CANINE AND FELINE
NUTRITION AND DIETETICS
A guide for the general practitioner

Debora Guidi

CANINE AND FELINE
NUTRITION
AND DIETETICS
A guide for the general practitioner

In collaboration with
Raimondo Colangeli

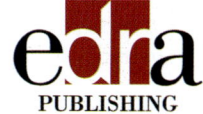

Authors

Debora Guidi
DVM, Resident ECVCN
Department of Veterinary Sciences, Università degli Studi di Torino

Raimondo Colangeli
DVM, Expert in Behavioral medicine
Vicepresident ANMVI (Associazione Nazionale Medici Veterinari Italiani)
Past President SISCA (Società Italiana Scienze del Comportamento Animale)

The Authors would like to thank for their contribution:

Alessia Candellone
DVM, EMSAVM, PHD
Department of Veterinary Sciences, Università degli Studi di Torino

Natalia Russo
DVM, Resident ECVCN
Department of Veterinary Sciences, Università degli Studi di Torino

Diana Vergnano
DVM, Dipl. ECVCN
Department of Veterinary Sciences, Università degli Studi di Torino

Foreword

I am pleased to write the foreword of this text by Debora Guidi, since veterinary nutrition, the discipline to which it is dedicated, is the passion that we both share and that led us to know each other almost 15 years ago. Doctor Guidi and I worked on the development and diffusion of veterinary nutrition when this discipline, in Italy, counted as many advocates as there are fingers on one hand.

In these 15 years we have together seen the enormous development that the discipline has had, but as often happens in periods of expansion, we have also witnessed the advent, on the market, of figures who address this science in a brief manner. Nutrition, of all medical specialties, is probably one of the most exact sciences and, as such, leaves very little room for the approximation and birth of different schools of thought.

Every day the owners of animals have the need to confront the veterinarian on the issue of nutrition, since feeding their own animal is a situation that is dealt with daily, from the moment that the animal is a puppy to the specific nutrition in pathological states. Today, all owners know how much nutrition is a key factor in both disease prevention and their management, therefore it is normal for them to expect to find an interlocutor who is up to the situation in their veterinarian. The aim of this book is precisely to provide the veterinarian with some evidence-based nutritional recommendations that go beyond "emotional" fashions and factors that sometimes, in addition to involving the owners, also involve the veterinarian.

Liviana Prola
DVM, ECVCN Dipl.
Department of Veterinary Sciences
Università degli Studi di Torino

Introduction

*Let food be thy medicine
and medicine be thy food.*
Hippocrates of Cos

To date, nutrition has never been the first of the recommendations to be taken into account in veterinary practice. Over the years, however, it has been understood how important it is, especially in healthy animals, to maintain a good state of health, prolong the average life and prevent the onset of diseases such as obesity, diabetes mellitus, liver lipidosis etc.

The aim of this volume is to give nutritional advice which can be used in daily practice, to provide simple answers to the most frequently asked questions of our customers and to the needs of our patients, seeking the right compromise between knowledge and practicality. It starts with an overview of the basic nutrients and then we take into consideration nutrition at various stages of life, indicate which type of food to choose and how to compare the different foods, we evaluate the most correct nutritional approach for the most frequently diagnosed diseases.

The book also presents some simple recipes to be used in daily practice, together with the indications provided in the nutritional handbooks of different manufacturers of food, so that the customers can be able to choose and decide to choose the type of diet they want to follow. Finally, the chapter by Raimondo Colangeli deals with the theme of nutrition from a behavioral point of view, offering new and really useful food for thought in daily clinical practice.

Acknowledgments

It doesn't often happen to do a job that we like and that, at the same time, has always been our passion. It happened to me. This is what I thank my parents for, who have supported me during many difficulties, allowing me to become a veterinarian and to achieve what has been my biggest dream since my childhood.

I thank my sister Barbara, who has always been close to me and is a guide and a support for me.

I thank Liviana Prola for giving me the opportunity to follow and grow my second passion, that of the nutrition. I still remember the email I sent her requesting to embark on the long journey of the European Diploma with her, but I remember even clearly her answer and the great adventure that followed!

Finally, I thank my children Valerio, Marco and Gaia for their patience and their great support. I say to them: "I willed, and I always willed, and I willed passionately".

Table of contents

Chapter 1

Nutrients and nutritional needs

We are what we eat

OBJECTIVES OF THIS CHAPTER
• Knowing the nutrients and nutritional needs to avoid deficiencies or excesses • Calculate the daily needs and the energy density of the diet in order to plan a correct rationing

Dogs and cats are both mammals that belong to the order of carnivores, but the evolutionary history of dogs, indicates a more omnivorous natural diet than the diet of the cat, which has been carnivorous throughout its evolutionary path. In fact, we can define cats as a "strict carnivore", and dogs as an "adapted carnivore" or, even, an "opportunistic carnivore".

This can also be seen by examining their teeth: the two species have the same number of incisors and canines, but dogs has a higher number of molars and premolars, therefore they are able to chew and crush food better than cats. This type of dentition is probably linked to a higher intake of vegetable substances or, in general, to a more omnivorous diet.

In this chapter, we will examine the nutrients and the nutritional needs, as the knowledge of them allows us to answer another important question.

How much and what should a diet provide?

In addition to meeting the *energy needs*, the diet must supply the organism with *water*, *proteins*, *carbohydrates*, *fats*, *vitamins* and *minerals* (Figure 1.1). It is important to remember that no nutrient acts alone, but the interactions between different nutrients, are essential for the correct functioning of the whole organism. All these interactions occur during absorption, usage and elimination.

In addition to knowing what nutrients are, it is also important to know their quantities.

Where can we find the reference quantities to avoid deficiencies or excesses?

The reference quantities are found in the tables of the AAFCO (Association of American Feed Control Officials), the NRC (National Research Council, Nutrient Requirement of Dogs and Cats) or the FEDIAF (European Pet Food Industry Federation). The latter are those that we use and they are easily available online, for free (www.fediaf.org).

All the nutrient values are reported for both cats and dogs, when adults or in the growth phase, in order to provide a complete and balanced diet for them.

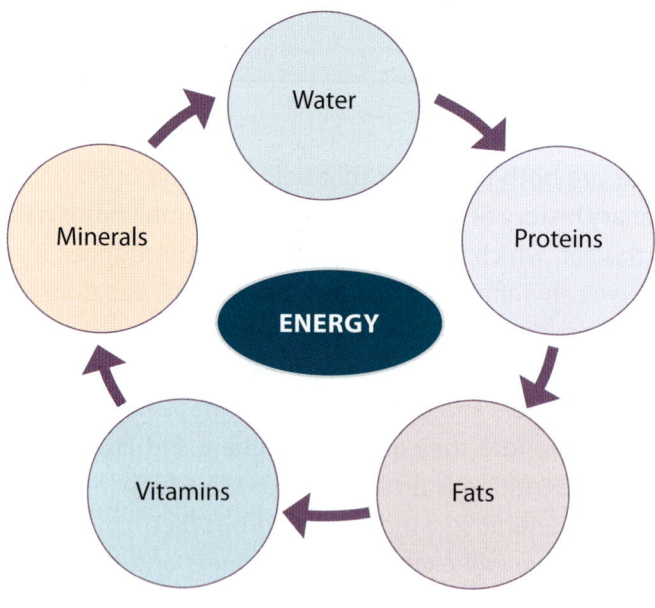

■ **FIGURE 1.1** Nutritional principles.

However, be careful: it is important to know that those indicated are minimum values, and we shouldn't go below them, to avoid deficiencies. Some maximum nutritional and legal values are also reported. Nutritional values are the maximum levels which, according to recent studies, have not been associated with harmful effects: overcoming them may not be harmful, but since there are no studies on this topic, it is advisable to avoid it. The legal values, however, are regulated and reported in an additives register (1831/2003/EC); referring to some minerals and vitamin D when they are added precisely as additives to recipes, therefore it is mandatory not to exceed them.

The digestive systems of dogs and cats are very different from that of other pets and from humans. The biggest difference is in the length of the intestine: while the bovine intestine is about 20 times the length of the body, that of a horse 12 times and a pig 14 times, a dog's intestine is five times the length of it's body and a cat's intestine, only four times. The intestine of these animals, therefore, is short and the digestive processes are very rapid, so it is important to provide them with high quality and highly digestible foods. In order to better digest and assimilate food, dogs should eat 2-3 times a day. Cats, on the other hand, should eat little portions often.

Eating only once a day not only creates problems in the digestion of the food, with the appearance of diarrhea and deficiencies, but can also predispose dogs to gastric dilatation and torsion, and cats to problems with the lower urinary tract.

Water

Water is the most important nutrient for life. 60-75% of an organism's body weight is made of water. An animal can survive after losing almost all its fat and more than half its proteins, but if it loses about 10% of its body water, it can face death. The supply of water for domestic carnivores, as well as in humans and other animals, is fundamental not only because it is the main constituent, indispensable for all metabolic processes and exchanges that take place in the body, but also because water helps to adjust the body temperature.

Animals take water both directly and through food and lose it with urine, feces and perspiration. The need for water is of a critical importance especially when the temperature is high, when the animal works intensely, when there is a strong loss through milk, feces (diarrhea), urine or blood (hemorrhage).

Animals must always have fresh and drinking water to drink, free of unpleasant smells and tastes, at a temperature of about 10-25° C.

Of course, it is also important to regularly check the hygienic conditions of the water containers.

 Above all, it is essential for cats to take water through food, therefore the food is preferably wet or especially moist.

Energy

Energy is the body's fuel and is derived from proteins, fats and carbohydrates. Energy is used to maintain a constant body temperature, to make the various organs and tissues work, for growth, milk production and muscles work. Only a part of the ingested energy is used (about 75%) and it is called metabolizable energy (ME); the rest is lost in feces and urine (Figure 1.2).

The various nutrients (proteins, fats and carbohydrates) provide different amounts of metabolizable energy. Fats are the most efficient, and it is important to keep this in mind, especially in the context of the low-calorie diets. Sometimes the energy density of a food is shown on the package; otherwise, it can be determined in different ways, one of which is the multiplication of the amount of proteins, fats and carbohydrates contained in the food by some values (respectively 3.5; 8.5; 3.5 kcal) called modified Atwater factors. Energy density is measured in kilocalories (kcal) or joules (J) (Table 1.1).

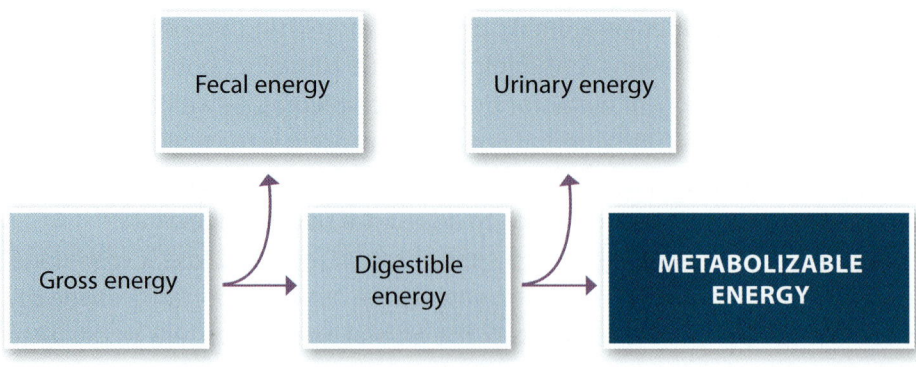

FIGURE 1.2 Metabolizable energy.

■ **TABLE 1.1 - MODIFIED ATWATER FACTORS**

Nutrients*	Kilocalories
Carbohydrates	3.5
Lipids	8.5
Proteins	3.5

*In 1 g of food.

In addition to the energy density of a food, it is also important to determine the daily energy needs of an animal, since it affects the quantities of food taken and, consequently, those of the other nutrients. The variables that can change the maintenance of needs are numerous, for example the temperature, age, physiological state and the physical activity. In addition, in the canine species there is an extreme inhomogeneity between individuals, which is unseen in other species. Weight variations range from 1 to 100 kg; the coat can be long and thick or almost absent; the nature, and consequently spontaneous physical activity, is very different. For this reason, the energy needed by the body is related to the body surface and not to the weight, and in this case we speak of metabolic weight.

A dog's maintenance energy requirement (MER) can be calculated in several ways. The most used formula is the following one:

$$MER = 110 \times (weight\ in\ kg)^{0.75}$$

If necessary, then, correction factors can be applied by multiplying them by the MER (Table 1.2).

MER is defined as the energy requirement of an adult animal with moderate physical activity in the conditions of thermoneutrality (25° C for short-haired animals, 14° C for long-haired ones).

There are also several ways to calculate the MER for cats. Those that we use are:

$$MER = 70 \times (weight\ in\ kg)^{0.75}$$
$$MER = 70 \times (weight\ in\ kg)^{0.75} \times 0.8\ (if\ sterilized/neutered)$$

The determination of the energy density of the food and the animal's energy needs is the real key to rationing. Through a simple proportion we can determine and then indicate the quantity of food to be administered daily (Figure 1.3).

■ TABLE 1.2 - CORRECTION FACTORS FOR CALCULATING THE MER

Age	1-2 years	× 1.10
Temperature	30-35° C	× 1.2
	20° C	× 1
	<10° C	× 1.1 (except Nordic breeds)
	<0° C	× 1.2 (except Nordic breeds)
	−10° C	× 1.5
Activity and temperament	Normal-moderate	× 1.2
	Nervous-active	× 1.3
Race	Nordic or predisposed to obesity (Beagle, Labrador, Golden Retriever, Cocker, Boxer etc.)	× 0.9
	Predisposed to underweight. (Greyhounds, Great Danes etc.)	× 1.1

Dog: required 1,000 kcal/day

Food: 400 kcal/day

How much should be taken per day?

400 kcal : 100 g = 1,000 kcal : x g

x = 100 x 1,000 / 400 = **250 g/day**

■ FIGURE 1.3 Example of determining the amount of food to be administered daily to a dog.

All these formulas must be a starting point. It is important to constantly monitor the weight of the animal, in order to increase or decrease the calories if necessary. We always recommend starting with a minimum/basic requirement: our pets rarely have a high energy expenditure.

Proteins

Proteins are complex molecules. They can be divided into simple proteins if they are made up only of amino acids, such as plasma albumin, milk lactalbumin, corn zein and the structural proteins, keratin, collagen and elastin, and in complex proteins if they are made up of amino acids and non-protein molecules, such as nucleoproteins, glycoproteins and phosphoproteins.

Proteins perform numerous functions in the body and are the main constituents of hair, feathers, ligaments, tendons, muscles etc. They carry out numerous metabolic reactions and are essential for digestion, absorption etc. They have different hormonal functions, for example insulin and glucagon, or transport proteins, such as hemoglobin (for oxygen) and transferrin (for iron). They are important for the acid-base balance of the body and are the main constituents of the immune system, the antibodies.

The main constituents of proteins are amino acids, which are divided into essential and non-essential (Table 1.3). The essential amino acids must be supplied with the diet because they cannot be synthesized by the body. In dogs there are 10 essential amino acids; the most important are arginine, methionine, tryptophan and lysine. There are 11 in cats, because there is also the well-known taurine.

Proteins are constantly demolished and synthesized; in fact, the body is able to synthesize new ones if the essential amino acids and nitrogen are present, but it is not able to preserve them.

Proteins, if supplied in quantities, greater than the needs, are used for energy purposes or transformed into fats and carbohydrates.

■ **TABLE 1.3 - ESSENTIAL AND NON-ESSENTIAL AMINO ACIDS**

Essential amino acids	Non-essential amino acids
Arginine	Alanine
Histidine	Asparagine
Isoleucine	Aspartic acid
Leucine	Cysteine
Lysine	Glutaminic acid
Methionine	Glutamine
Phenylalanine	Glycine
Tryptophan	Hydroxylysine
Threonine	Hydroxyproline
Valine	Proline
Taurine (cats)	Serine
	Tyrosine

The determination of the protein requirement for our pets is not easy to establish, since it depends on numerous factors such as quality, amino acid composition and digestibility; in addition, the energy density of the diet, the age and the degree of activity of the animal, also directly influence the needs of the individual. Cats have a significantly higher protein requirement than that of dogs, due to several factors including a greater need for essential amino acids. This is evident especially in kittens, in which over 60% of the proteins are used for maintenance and only 40% for growth. The exact opposite occurs in dogs.

The following are the minimum protein requirements for adult dogs and cats (Tables 1.4 and 1.5), growing and reproducing (Tables 1.6 and 1.7).

▦ TABLE 1.4 - MINIMUM NEED FOR PROTEINS IN ADULT DOGS*

Adult MER 110 kcal/kg$^{0.75}$	18.00 g

*FEDIAF (2017), Unit per 100 g on the dry substance.

▦ TABLE 1.5 - MINIMUM NEED FOR PROTEINS IN ADULT CATS*

Adult MER 100 kcal/kg$^{0.67}$	25.00 g

*FEDIAF (2017), Unit per 100 g on the dry substance.

▦ TABLE 1.6 - MINIMUM NEED FOR PROTEINS IN DOG'S GROWTH AND REPRODUCTION*

First phase of growth (<14 weeks) Reproduction	25.00 g
Second phase of growth (≥14 weeks) Reproduction	20.00 g

*FEDIAF (2017), Unit per 100 g on the dry substance.

▦ TABLE 1.7 - MINIMUM NEED OF PROTEIN IN CAT'S GROWTH AND REPRODUCTION*

Growth/Reproduction	28.00/30.00 g

*FEDIAF (2017), Unit per 100 g on the dry substance.

 Protein sources that can be used, are meat, fish, eggs, soy and legumes. Vegetable proteins are not balanced and available/digestible like high quality animal proteins, but they are superior to those contained in poor quality animal derivatives such as bones, heads, legs etc.

Obviously, the essential amino acids are all important, but here we will focus in particular on taurine and arginine.

Taurine

Taurine is found as a free amino acid in animal tissues, while it is completely absent in the plant world. Meat, poultry, fish, shellfish (and mice!) are particularly rich in it. In most mammals it can be synthesized from methionine and cysteine, but not in cats (Figure 1.4). Furthermore, since cats have a much higher need than the other animals, it is very sensitive to its deficiency in the diet.

Taurine deficiency involves a series of alterations in the reproductive activity, especially in females, in the conjugation of bile acids – with a decrease in the absorption of vitamins and fats, alterations of the retina (central degeneration of the retina) with loss of vision – and of the heart (dilated cardiomyopathy), with a decrease in muscle contractility and heart failure.

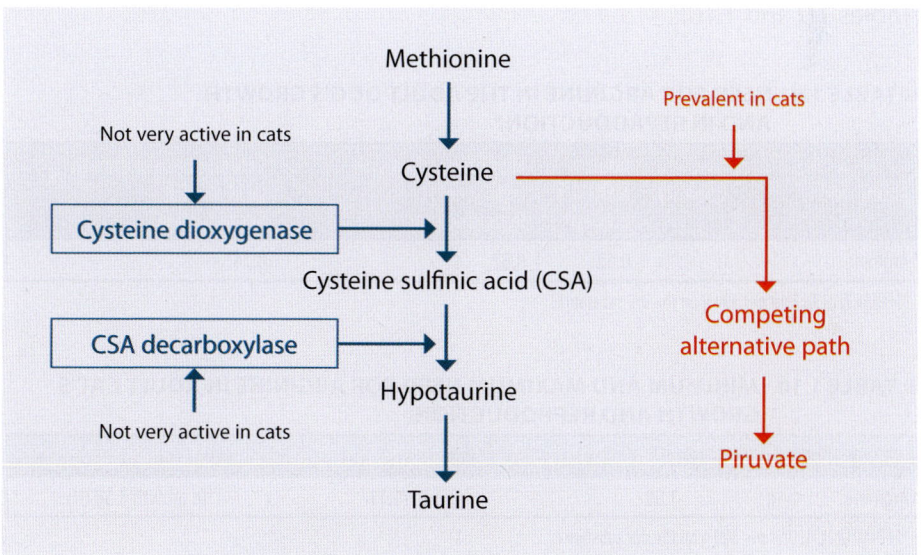

FIGURE 1.4 Metabolic pathway of taurine synthesis.

▤ TABLE 1.8 - TAURINE NEED IN THE ADULT CAT'S GROWTH AND IN REPRODUCTION*

Amino acid	Quantity	Adult MER 100 kcal/kg$^{0.67}$	Growth and reproduction
Taurine (wet food)	g	0.20	0.25
Taurine (dry food)	g	0.10	0.10

*FEDIAF (2017), Unit per 100 g on the dry substance.

The required amount of taurine changes according to the type of food, as its degradation by bacterial flora varies. In wet foods the integrated quantity must be greater, to avoid possible deficiencies (Table 1.8).

Arginine

Arginine is an essential amino acid and it is necessary for the organism, for protein synthesis and for the urea cycle. This substance allows the conversion of ammonia produced by the metabolism of proteins, in urea, which is then eliminated. The absence of arginine in food causes an immediate and serious deficiency. Cats can develop severe hyperammonemia even within hours of eating a protein meal. Symptoms include vomiting, muscle spasms, ataxia, tetanus spasms, until coma and death.

Dogs may also exhibit these symptoms, but in a less severe form. The importance of arginine for the urea cycle, associated with high protein catabolism which is not very flexible, makes the cat much more sensitive to its deficiency (Tables 1.9 and 1.10).

▤ TABLE 1.9 - NEED FOR ARGININE IN THE ADULT DOG'S GROWTH AND IN REPRODUCTION*

Amino acid	Quantity	Adult MER 110 kcal/kg$^{0.75}$	First phase of growth (<14 weeks) Reproduction	Second phase of growth (≥14 weeks) Reproduction
Arginine	g	0.52	0.82	0.74

*FEDIAF (2017), Unit per 100 g on the dry substance.

▤ TABLE 1.10 - MINIMUM AND MAXIMUM NEED FOR ARGININE IN ADULT CAT'S GROWTH AND REPRODUCTION*

Amino acid	Quantity	Adult MER 100 kcal/kg$^{0.67}$	Growth and reproduction	Maximum quantity
Arginine	g	1.00	1.07/1.11	In growth 3.50 (N)

*FEDIAF (2017), Unit per 100 g on the dry substance.
N = nutritional.

Arginine deficiency can also be relative. The higher the protein level, the higher its concentration.

In dogs, 0.1 g more arginine must be supplied for every 1% extra protein. In cats, 0.2 g more arginine for every 1% extra protein.

Fats

Fats, or lipids, perform numerous functions in the body. They are the primary source of energy, regulate thermogenesis, are the transporters of fat-soluble vitamins and provide essential fatty acids. Fats have a high energy content (8.5 kcal/g of metabolizable energy) and a very high digestibility (>90%). Carnivores, thanks to the conspicuous biliary secretion, have a high ability to use them, therefore fats can constitute up to 15-30% of the daily ration.

The simplest and most abundant lipids in nature are triglycerides. These are the main source of food lipids and the main "fuels" for most organisms. They represent the most important form of chemical energy reserve.

The main constituents of lipids are fatty acids, which differ from each other in the length of the chain (4-24 carbon atoms) and in the presence, number and position of their double bonds (saturated, monounsaturated, polyunsaturated).

Two families of fatty acids are very important for the body, those of the omega-6 and omega-3 series (ω-6, ω-3). Among the most important fatty acids of the omega-6 series, we find linoleic acid (essential fatty acid for both cats and dogs), gamma linolenic acid and arachidonic acid (essential fatty acids for cats and puppies). Among those in the omega-3 series we find alpha-linolenic acid, docosahexaenoic acid (DHA) and eicosapentaenoic acid (EPA).

The fat of terrestrial animals is very rich in omega-6 series fatty acids, while that of marine animals is rich in omega-3 series.

Essential fatty acids (EFA) cannot be produced by the body, therefore they must be taken with the diet like the essential amino acids (Figure 1.5; Tables 1.11 and 1.12). The lack of EFA, in particular of the linoleic acid, leads to alterations of the skin and coat: opaque and dry hair, alopecia, skin lesions, scaling, interdigital exudation, otitis. The adult dog, like most animals, is able to synthesize the fatty acids of the omega-6 series starting from linoleic acid.

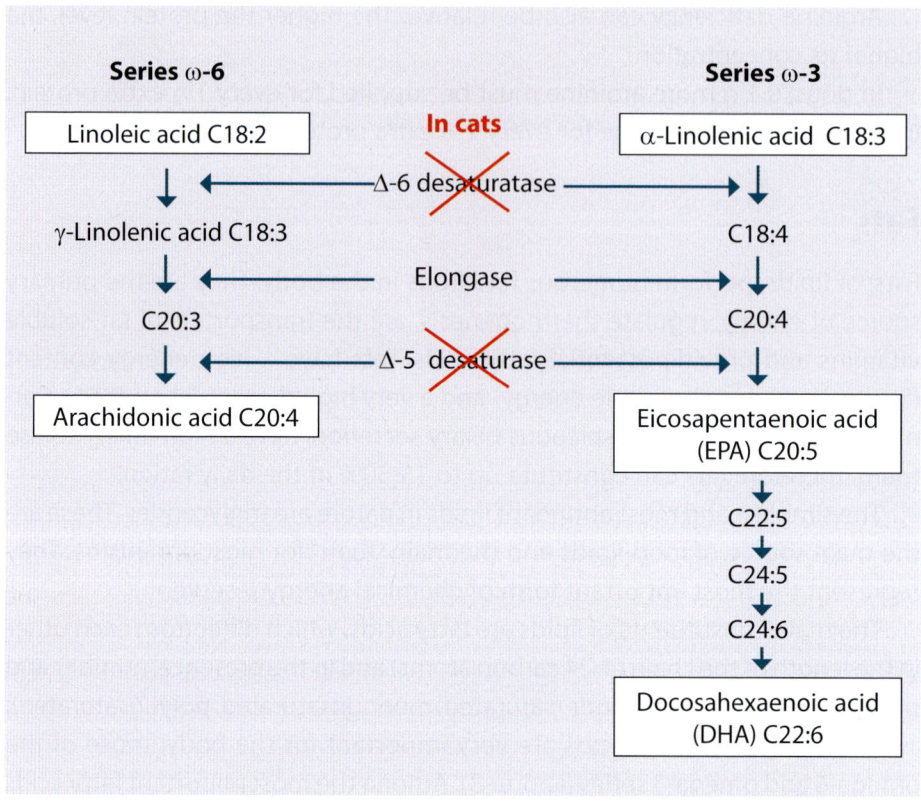

FIGURE 1.5 Metabolic pathway of omega-6 and omega-3 fatty acid synthesis.

TABLE 1.11 - MINIMUM AND MAXIMUM NEEDS FOR FATS AND FATTY ACIDS IN ADULT DOG'S GROWTH AND REPRODUCTION*

Fats and fatty acids	Quantity	Adult MER 110 kcal/kg$^{0.75}$	First phase of growth (<14 weeks) reproduction	Second phase of growth (<14 weeks) reproduction	Maximum quantity
Fats	g	5.50	8.50	8.50	–
Linoleic acid	g	1.32	1.30	1.30	First phase of growth 6.50 (N)
Arachidonic acid	mg	–	30.00	30.00	–
α-Linolenic acid	g	–	0.08	0.08	–
EPA + DHA	g	–	0.05	0.05	–

*FEDIAF (2017), Unit per 100 g on the dry substance.
N = nutritional.

■ **TABLE 1.12 - MINIMUM NEED FOR FAT AND FATTY ACIDS IN ADULT CAT'S GROWTH AND REPRODUCTION***

Fats and fatty acids	Quantity	Adult MER 100 kcal/kg$^{0.67}$	Growth and reproduction
Fats	g	9.00	9.00
Linoleic acid	g	0.50	0.55
Arachidonic acid	mg	6.00	20.00
α-Linolenic acid	g	–	0.02
EPA + DHA	g	–	0.01

*FEDIAF (2017), Unit per 100 g on the dry substance.

Cats and puppies, on the other hand, are not capable synthetizing it, therefore they also need a food intake of arachidonic acid. The deficiency of this fatty acid involves the development of an alteration of blood coagulation (alteration of platelet aggregation and thrombocytopenia) and an alteration of reproductive capacity. Arachidonic acid is present only in animal tissues and this is further confirmation of the fact that the cat is a strict carnivore. DHA and EPA are essential in growth: their deficiency leads to insufficient development of the nervous system, retina and acoustic nerve.

EFA deficiencies are however rare and require a long period to manifest. They are often linked to poorly formulated or incorrectly stored diets; in fact, high temperatures and humidity can promote rancidity and therefore the loss of these substances. Furthermore, EFAs can be inactivated even when the level of antioxidants in the diet is insufficient (for example with a lack of vitamins E and C). We have seen how EFA deficiency leads to serious problems, especially dermatological problems, due to the high turnover of skin cells, with dry skin, dull hair, alopecia, itching, skin lesions and secondary infections, but also an excessive lipid intake can determine various problems, such as weight gain, obesity, diarrhea etc. Not only their presence, but also the ratio between omega-6 and omega-3 fatty acids is very important, especially in allergic animals (5:1/3:1). It has long been proven that the increase in omega-3 in the diet, is fundamental in the treatment of inflammatory dermatitis and many other diseases.

Fats that can be used in the diet are olive oil, sunflower oil, peanut oil, fish oil, chicken fat, pork fat etc.

Carbohydrates

Carbohydrates are the main energy components of plants and make up 60-90% of the dry matter. They can be divided into (1) monosaccharides, simple sugars such as glucose, fructose and galactose; (2) disaccharides, such as lactose (glucose + galactose), present in the milk of all mammals, or sucrose (glucose + fructose), known as table sugar (Box 1.1); (3) polysaccharides such as starch, glycogen, dextrins and fibers (cellulose, hemicellulose, pectin, rubber and mucilage) (Figure 1.6).

BOX 1.1 DISACCHARIDES

Some disaccharides, such as sucrose or lactose, are not well tolerated by dogs and cats. This depends on the digestive enzymes present: if they are very low or absent, sometimes there may be diarrhea related to the osmotic effect of sugar which escapes digestion and the excessive production of volatile fatty acids by bacteria.

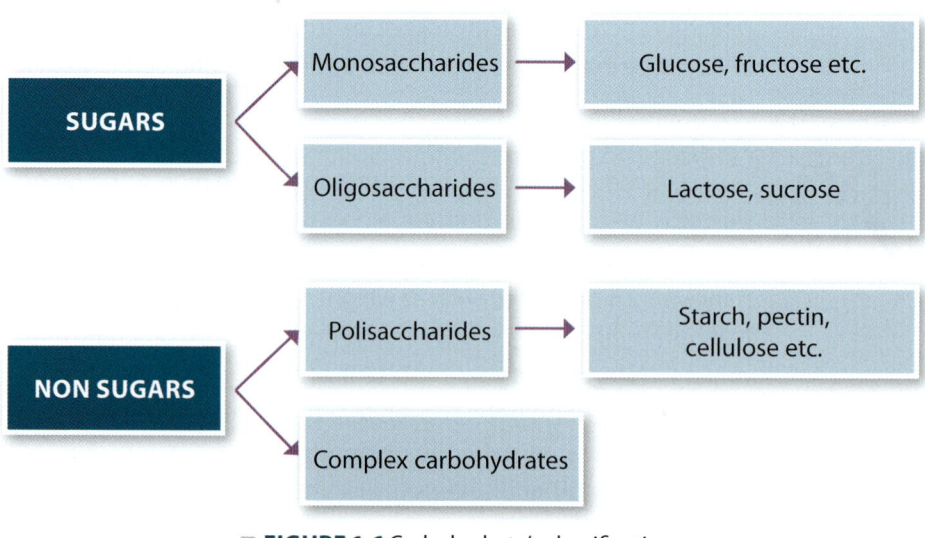

■ **FIGURE 1.6** Carbohydrate's classification.

Carbohydrates are important for several reasons: they provide the carbon structure for the synthesis, for example, of amino acids, DNA and RNA, they are an important source of energy, they are indispensable for the proper functioning of the gastrointestinal system (fibers) and, conjugated together with proteins or lipids, become structural components of the tissues.

All animals have a metabolic need for carbohydrates and this need can be met with endogenous production, using proteins, in particular glucogenic amino acids (alanine, glycine, serine etc.), or glycerol, or with direct food intake of carbohydrates.

When this need increases as the animal grows, during pregnancy (for fetal development) and during breastfeeding (for the synthesis of lactose), an adequate presence of carbohydrates or their precursors in the diet is necessary to maintain normal metabolic processes. In these situations, carbohydrates become "necessary in a conditional way" and we recommend the presence of at least 20% in the diet.

Starch is the main carbohydrate present in food. Cereals such as corn, wheat and rice are its main sources. The potato is also rich in starch and therefore it is frequently used.

Starch is an important economic energy source for the extrusion process (croquettes). Once cooked, it is digested by both cats and dogs, and this allows the body to save proteins, which are therefore used for other purposes.

Carbohydrates include fiber, which is very important for our pets. Based on their chemical-physical characteristics and their relationship with water, they contribute in various ways to the proper functioning of the gastrointestinal system, promoting intestinal peristalsis, increasing or decreasing the absorption of nutrients, increasing local immune defenses and digestion of nutrients. They can be divided into soluble, insoluble or viscous, or rapidly, medium or non-fermentable (Table 1.13; Figure 1.7). It is important to know them in order to make the best use of them.

The more soluble and fermentable the fibers, the more intestinal transit and fecal mass decrease, while the acid excretion of bile increases. The more the quantity of fiber, which is able to retain water, the more the fecal volume increases. All the fibers retain more or less water, but the insoluble and medium fermentable ones generally do so to a greater extent (for example cellulose). Some are able to form viscous solutions and gels that reduce absorption, postprandial blood glucose, gastric emptying and transit in the caecum, properties evidently useful in some pathologies (for example diabetes mellitus). They are less useful or contraindicated in other pathologies (for example gastritis).

■ **TABLE 1.13 - CARBOHYDRATES AND THEIR FERMENTABILITY CHARACTERISTICS AND SOLUBILITY**

Starches, sugars and fiber	Fermentability	Solubility
Fructans, galactans, mannans, mucillages	Quickly fermentable	Soluble
Pectin	Quickly and on average fermentable	Soluble
Hemicellulose	Medium and slowly fermentable	Soluble and insoluble
Cellulose	Slowly fermentable	Insoluble
Lignin	Not digestible or fermentable	–
Resistant starches	Moderately fermentable	–
Starches	Enzymatically digested	–
Mono- and disaccharides	Absorbed	–

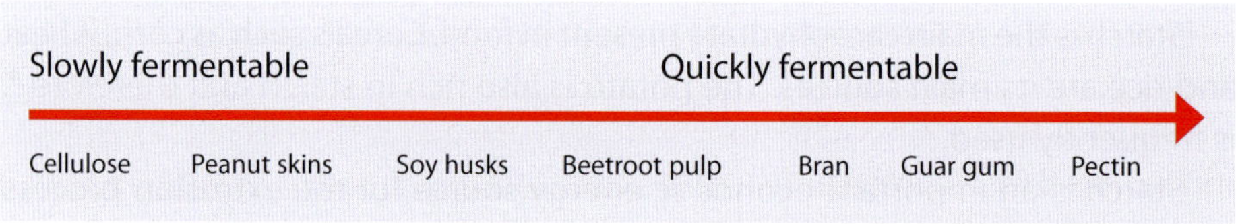

Slowly fermentable   Quickly fermentable

Cellulose   Peanut skins   Soy husks   Beetroot pulp   Bran   Guar gum   Pectin

■ **FIGURE 1.7** Carbohydrates: from the least to the most fermentable.

These fibers also seem very useful in promoting the transit of cat hairballs, reducing the phenomena of chronic vomiting. Fibers with these characteristics are: *psyllium*, pea or oat fiber, beet pulp.

In the last 10 years, much attention has been paid to prebiotic fibers, which have different levels of solubility and fermentability and are capable of supporting the growth of the "good" intestinal bacterial flora (bifidobacteria, lactobacilli) at the expense of the pathogenic one (*Bacteroides* and *Clostridium* spp.).

Furthermore, the fermentation of these fibers leads to the formation of short chain fatty acids (SCFA), which reduce the intestinal pH and inhibit the growth of pathogenic bacteria, and nourish the intestine (acetate, propinate or butyrate). Butyrate is preferentially used by the cells of the intestine, particularly the colon. It has been seen that this leads to an increase in the number of colonocytes, the weight of the intestinal mucosa, the absorption of water and electrolytes and the activity of digestive enzymes, and a reduction in adhesion and bacterial translocation.

Among the prebiotic fibers, the most known and studied ones are the fruit-oligosaccharides (FOS) and the mannan-ooligosaccharides (MOS).

Speaking of prebiotics we should not forget to mention the *probiotics*. The term probiotics refers to live and viable bacteria which, when taken, have beneficial effects on the host. They must be able to resist the acidic environment of the stomach and bile and must be able to adhere and / or multiply in the intestinal tract. There are studies that demonstrate various beneficial effects of these microorganisms (immunomodulators, anti-inflammatories, antiallergics, anticancer agents, antidiarrheal agents) at concentrations of 1×10^8-1×10^{11} of colony-forming units per day (CFU/day), especially in humans. There are not many studies done for cats and dogs, for the most part, they are not decisive.

Vitamins

Vitamins are organic molecules needed in small quantities and are indispensable for the growth and survival of all living beings, in obviously different quantities depending on the species and physiological state. They are present in some foods and absent in others. The term vitamin was coined only in 1912 and is linked to the importance of these substances for life.

One of the first reports of vitamin deficiency dates back to 2600 B.C.E. and it concerns beriberi, a disease that affected the nervous system of people who mainly ate polished rice, free of vitamin B_1. Scurvy, due to a deficiency of vitamin C, was known to the Egyptians from 1500 B.C.E.

Most vitamins are not synthesized by the organism, therefore they must be taken along with the diet. They are divided into *fat-soluble* and *water-soluble* vitamins. The first group includes vitamins A, D, E, K. In the second group we find the complex of vitamins B and vitamin C. Fat-soluble vitamins can be accumulated in the body, therefore they can have a potential toxicity. However, for the same reason, their deficiency is less common and develops more slowly (Table 1.14).

The food sources of vitamins are meat, fish, milk, eggs, leafy vegetables, citrus fruits, legumes etc.

Each vitamin has its own mechanism of action and when it is deficient, there are typical manifestations. Even an excessive intake of vitamins can cause serious breakdowns and pathologies. Today, in fact, the biggest problems are due to excessive intake. Obviously all vitamins are important, but we will mention only some of them below.

■ TABLE 1.14 - VITAMINS: FUNCTIONS AND SYMPTOMS OF DEFICIENCY

Vitamins	Functions	Symptoms of deficiency
A	Protects epithelia, controls growth and reproduction	Inflammation of the conjunctiva, poor growth
D	Anti-rickets, regulates the absorption of calcium and phosphorus	Rickets
E	Prevents muscular dystrophies and disorders of the reproductive system	Sterility and muscular dystrophies
K	Antihemorrhagic	Hemorrhage
B_1 (thiamine)	Regulates carbohydrate metabolism	Paralysis, convulsions, loss of appetite
B_2 (riboflavin)	Regulates the metabolism of amino acids and fats	Fatty infiltration of the liver, weight loss
B_6 (pyridoxine)	Regulates the metabolism of proteins, fats and carbohydrates	Weight loss, paralysis, anemia
PP (B_3, niacin)	Ensures the integrity of the skin and digestive system	Skin diseases, digestive tract disorders
B_{12} (cobalamin)	Participates in the formation of red blood cells	Growth retardation, anemia
H (B_8, biotin)	Keeps skin and coat in good condition	Dermatitis, depigmentation and hair loss
Pantothenic acid (B_5)	Controls growth, ensures good condition of skin and hair	Poor growth and hair loss
Folic acid (B_9)	Participates in the synthesis of hemoglobin	Anemia

Vitamin A

It occurs in several chemical forms, of which retinol is the most biologically active. It is important for the integrity of the epithelial tissue, for the skeleton, the reproductive system and for the eyes. Vitamin A can be found in milk, egg yolk and, in high quantities, in the liver.

In many animals, including humans and dogs, but not cats, it can be synthesized from some precursors, such as beta-carotene, which are found in some vegetables such as carrots, sweet potatoes or dark green vegetables. In cats, the intestinal enzyme capable of transforming carotenoids into vitamin A is strongly deficient or even absent, therefore it is more predisposed to deficiencies and must be fed with animal sources that contain this vitamin (strict carnivore). Vitamin A deficiency in young animals can lead to bone growth abnormalities and neurological disorders.

In adults there are changes in the reproductive and visual systems, in the skin and mucous epithelium of the gastrointestinal and, respiratory systems.

The most frequent symptoms are: anorexia, xerophthalmia, conjunctivitis, corneal opacity and ulcerations, skin lesions etc.

Like all fat-soluble vitamins, vitamin A can also be stored in the body, but precisely for this reason it can give problems, if taken in excessive quantities. Once again, the cat is the most sensitive, which can face a pathology, called deforming cervical spondylosis. In practice, bone neoformations develop at the cervical level which cause difficulty in movement, lameness and paralysis, in the most serious cases. In the past, these poisonings were more frequent, since there was a habit of feeding cats only with liver and milk. Today the use of a complete and balanced dedicated diet makes the onset of both deficiencies and intoxications with vitamin A very difficult.

Vitamin E

Also this vitamin is presented in different forms, of which the most active is alpha-tocopherol. It is a powerful antioxidant that protects the cell membranes of the body, blocking the oxidation (peroxidation) of lipids (phospholipids) by free radicals.

Vitamin E deficiency is not frequent, but it can be linked to poor food pre-servation or excessive integration with polyunsaturated fatty acids (PUFA). In dogs, vitamin E deficiency has been associated with skeletal muscle degenera-tion, reproductive problems, retinal degeneration, reduced immune response.

In cats it is linked with pansteatitis, characterized by edema of the deposited fat, anorexia, depression, fever, reluctance to movement, etc.

The food sources which are the richest in vitamin E are soybean oil, sunflo-wer oil, corn oil and wheat sprouts. Vitamin E is also present in fair quantities in nuts, green leafy vegetables, seeds etc.

Vitamin D

It includes a group of sterols which are present as provitamins, vitamin D_2 (ergocalciferol) and vitamin D_3 (cholecalciferol), which is of greater nutritional importance for the omnivores and carnivores. It can be either synthesized by the body when 7-dehydrocolecalciferol, a compound which is present in the skin, is exposed to sunlight, or taken with food; this way is the best for cats and dogs, as activation through the skin is poor.

Vitamin D is involved in a complex way in the homeostasis of calcium and phosphorus. Its effect is expressed on the intestine, bone and kidney, resulting in an increase in calcium and phosphorus to levels which are necessary for mineralization and bone remodeling. Its shortage determines an alteration of mineralization, causing rickets in puppies and osteomalacia in adults. Hyper-vitaminosis D causes bone demineralization, lameness, fractures, calcium deposits in the heart, kidney and large blood vessels.

Vitamin D is contained in moderate quantities in egg yolk and liver.

Minerals

Minerals are very important inorganic elements for the body's metabolic processes. They can be divided into macroelements, present in large quantities in the body, such as calcium, phosphorus, magnesium, sulfur, sodium, potassium, chlorine, and in microelements, which are present in traces or in very low concentrations, such as zinc, manganese, iodine etc.

They perform numerous functions and are often linked to each other, such as calcium and phosphorus, and this can influence their absorption, metabolism, the same activity etc. Other important relationships are those between calcium and magnesium or between zinc and calcium.

As we have already seen for other nutrients, nowadays the main problems are related to excesses or even imbalances caused by the interaction with other substances, such as phytates, which, if present in food, can alter, the absorption of iron, zinc and, to a lesser extent, also calcium and magnesium.

Table 1.15 summarizes the functions and symptoms related to the deficiency of various minerals. Below, we will analyze in detail two elements in particular, calcium and phosphorus.

■ TABLE 1.15 - MINERALS: FUNCTIONS AND SYMPTOMS OF DEFICIENCY

Minerals	Functions	Symptoms of deficiency
Calcium and phosphorus	Bone and tooth formation	Rickets in young puppies, osteoporosis in the elderly
Potassium	Control of nerve transmission and muscle functioning	Muscle weakness, heart and kidney injury
Chlorine and sodium	Electrolyte balance control	Fatigue, dry skin, hair loss
Magnesium	Bone formation	"Slipper" feet
Iron and copper	Formation of red blood cells, transport of oxygen	Weakness, anemia
Manganese	Ossification, control of reproductive functions	Poor growth, metabolic disorders
Zinc	Formation of important enzymes	Skin and hair problems
Iodine	Thyroid functioning	Goiter, skin and hair problems

Calcium and phosphorus

Calcium is the main inorganic component of the bone: 99% of it is found in the skeleton and only 1% is free. The level of calcaemia is maintained and regulated by homeostatic mechanisms (parathyroid hormone, calcitonin and vitamin D) and is independent of food intake. Calcium is essential for the bones, the transmission of the nerve impulse, cardiac and muscle contraction in general and for blood clotting.

Phosphorus, deposited in the skeletal system, is mostly linked to calcium, performs many functions and is involved in almost all metabolic processes. It is a constituent of DNA, RNA, ATP, membrane phospholipids etc.

Calcium deficiency, as well as phosphorus deficiency, leads to reduced growth, bone demineralization, spontaneous fractures, rickets and osteofibrosis.

Excess phosphorus can be complicated with a possible calcium deficiency (nutritional hyperparathyroidism).

An excess of calcium hinders the absorption of other minerals (P and Zn) and it is, particularly in young dogs of large breeds, a factor predisposing to disorders affecting the locomotor system (Tables 1.16 and 1.17).

■ **TABLE 1.16 - MINIMUM AND MAXIMUM NEEDS FOR CALCIUM AND PHOSPHORUS IN ADULT DOG'S GROWTH AND REPRODUCTION***

Minerals	Quantity	Adult MER 110 kcal/ kg$^{0.75}$	First phase of growth (<14 weeks) Reproduction	Second phase of growth (≥14 weeks) Reproduction	Maximum quantity
Calcium	g	0.50	1.00	0.80-1.00	Adult 2.5 (N) First phase of growth 1.60 (N) Second phase of growth 1.80 (N)
Phosphorus	g	0.40	0.90	0.70	Adult 1.60 (N)
Ca/P			1:1		Adult 2:1 (N) First phase of growth 1.6:1 (N) Second phase of growth 1.8:1 (N)

*FEDIAF (2017), Unit per 100 g on the dry substance.
N = nutritional.

■ TABLE 1.17 - MINIMUM AND MAXIMUM NEEDS FOR CALCIUM AND PHOSPHORUS IN ADULT CAT'S GROWTH AND REPRODUCTION*

Minerals	Quantity	Adult MER 100 kcal/ kg$^{0.67}$	Growth and reproduction	Maximum quantity
Calcium	g	0.59	1.00	–
Phosphorus	g	0.50	0.84	–
Ca/P		1:1		Adult 2:1 (N) In growth 1.5:1 (N)

*FEDIAF (2017). Unit per 100 g on the dry substance.
N = nutritional.

Puppies have both active and passive absorption of calcium in the intestine, unlike the adult, which is only active. For this reason they are more sensitive to excesses and can face pathologies more easily.

As we have seen, not only the individual quantities are important but also their relationship. The optimal ratio of calcium/phosphorus, for both the dog and the cat, is 1:1.

Antioxidants

Antioxidants are molecules capable of blocking free radicals. The activity, usefulness and, therefore, the benefits associated with these substances have been repeatedly demonstrated and ascertained, not only for humans but also for our four-legged friends. Free radicals are unstable atoms or molecules that cause various damage both to the nucleus (including DNA) and to the cell membrane.

Free radicals are responsible for numerous diseases: more than 50 diseases have been related to them, including Alzheimer's and Parkinson's disease, diabetes, rheumatoid arthritis, tumors, cardiovascular diseases etc. All cells can be involved.

When the number of free radicals exceeds the number of the antioxidant barrier, we enter what is called the oxidative stress, rightly considered the new killer of our century.

Antioxidant substances and molecules are different. Among the best known are vitamin C, vitamin E and bioflavonoids.

Fresh vegetables and plants, especially flowers, leaves, fruits, seeds and kernels, are very rich in bioflavonoids, as well as their derivatives. There are no studies on the quantities that can be used for our pets and, sometimes, there are even contraindications to their use, such as in the case of vitamin C (lower urinary tract diseases).

Chapter 2

Nutrition in the different stages of life

There is no single ideal diet for everyone

<table>
<tr><td align="center">OBJECTIVES OF THIS CHAPTER</td></tr>
<tr><td>

- Knowing the different needs of cats and dogs during the different stages of life
- Choosing the correct diet avoiding deficiencies and excesses

</td></tr>
</table>

Knowing what the nutritional needs of healthy animals are, is fundamental, since it allows us to choose the most suitable diet and makes us able to maintain the ideal weight and a good state of health. Even the average life of pets has lengthened, and this seems to be linked, above all, to proper nutrition.

It is important to pay attention during all periods of their life: *since puppies*, because "good foundations allow us to build strong buildings that last over the time"; *to adults*, because "maintenance" is also important; *to an elderly age*, because this is the most delicate period and it is even more important not to generalize, but to adapt the diet to the individual, reevaluating it frequently.

☞ What should we evaluate/do?

First of all, we must evaluate their nutritional needs based on their age, whether in reproduction stage or not. As mentioned in the first chapter, there are several guidelines. The guidelines we use the most are the FEDIAF guidelines. Here we find the nutritional profiles and the minimum quantities and, in some cases, also the maximum of proteins, fats, vitamins and minerals needed in puppies, adults and during their reproduction. This allows us to avoid deficiencies and excesses and to evaluate whether a food is complete, balanced and suitable for our pet.

The second step is to ensure the right energy supply. The goal is to maintain the ideal weight and the right ratio between lean mass and fat mass. For this purpose we can use the formulas shown in the previous chapter. In our structure, a balance must always be present and in all our patients we must always evaluate the BCS (Body Condition Score) and the MCS (Muscle Condition Score). The BCS is aimed at visually evaluating fat deposits by palpation and it has some points of reference which are the fossa of the flank, the ribs, the lumbar vertebrae and the bones of the pelvis. There are two scales: the best one is the one divided into 9 points, as it allows you to better evaluate the subjects that are at the limits of the values (Figure 2.1). Five is the perfect number! At this value, the animal is in great shape and the weight marked by the scale can be considered its ideal weight. If the score increases, it means that the animal is overweight/obese. On the contrary, if it decreases, it is underweight. For each passage from one number to another on the scale, we must consider an increase/decrease of 10-20% of the ideal weight. (Figure 2.2; Box 2.1).

The 9-point scale is divided as follows:
- Underweight:
    1. Coasts, lumbar vertebrae, pelvic bones and other bony prominences visible at a distance; indistinguishable body fat; evident loss of muscle mass.
    2. Easily visible ribs, lumbar vertebrae and pelvic bones; absence of palpable fat; other partially visible bony prominences; minimal loss of muscle mass.
    3. Ribs are easily palpable, sometimes visible; absence of palpable fat; visible lumbar vertebral tops; prominent pelvic bones; noticeable abdominal girdle, pronounced abdominal retraction.
- Ideal weight:
    4. Easily palpable ribs, with minimal adipose coating; abdominal girdle clearly distinguishable from above; noticeable abdominal retraction.
    5. Palpable ribs without excessive adipose coating; abdominal girdle distinguishable from above; abdominal retraction visible laterally.
- Overweight:
    6. Palpable ribs with slight adipose coating; abdominal girdle distinguishable from above but not evident; appreciable abdominal retraction.

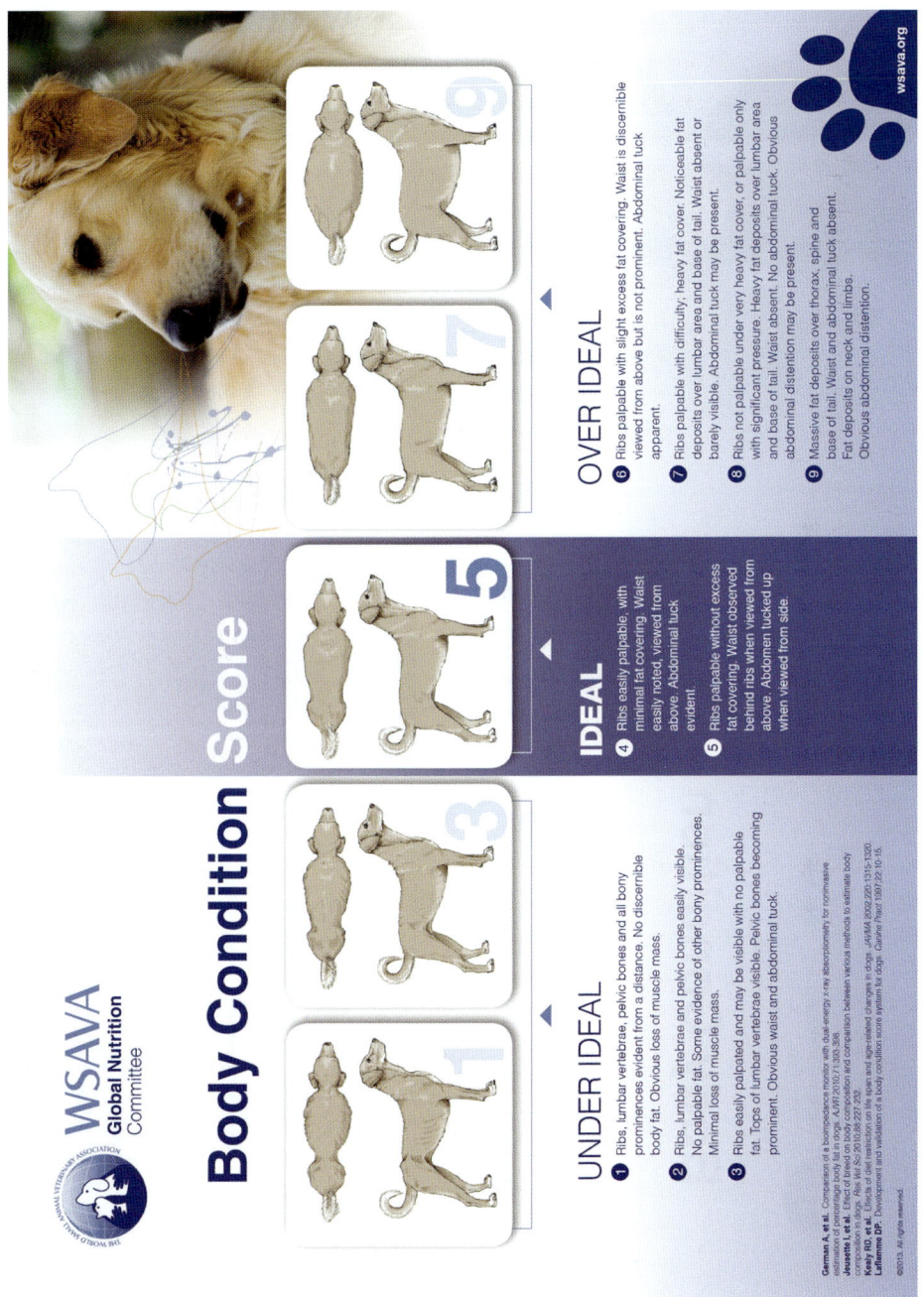

FIGURE 2.1 Body Condition Score (BCS). *Provided courtesy of the World Small Animal Veterinary Association (WSAVA). Available at the WSAVA Global Nutrition Committee Nutritional Toolkit website: https://www.wsava.org/Guidelines/Global-Nutrition-Guidelines. Accessed November 12, 2019. Copyright Tufts University, 2014.*

Continued on the next page

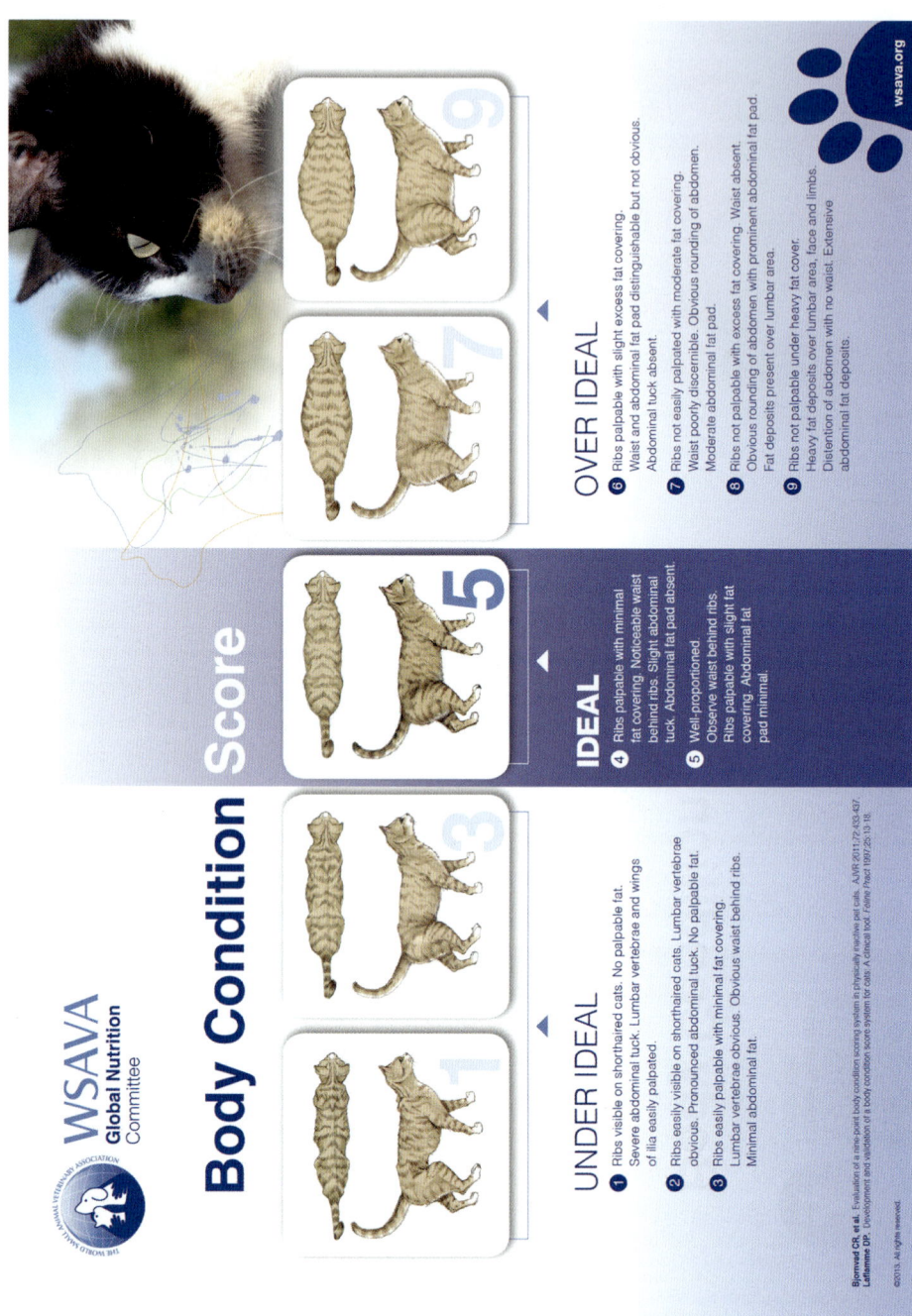

WSAVA
Global Nutrition
Committee

Body Condition Score

wsava.org

UNDER IDEAL

1. Ribs visible on shorthaired cats. No palpable fat. Severe abdominal tuck. Lumbar vertebrae and wings of ilia easily palpated.

2. Ribs easily visible on shorthaired cats. Lumbar vertebrae obvious. Pronounced abdominal tuck. No palpable fat.

3. Ribs easily palpable with minimal fat covering. Lumbar vertebrae obvious. Obvious waist behind ribs. Minimal abdominal fat.

IDEAL

4. Ribs palpable with minimal fat covering. Noticeable waist behind ribs. Slight abdominal tuck. Abdominal fat pad absent.

5. Well-proportioned. Observe waist behind ribs. Ribs palpable with slight fat covering. Abdominal fat pad minimal.

OVER IDEAL

6. Ribs palpable with slight excess fat covering. Waist and abdominal fat pad distinguishable but not obvious. Abdominal tuck absent.

7. Ribs not easily palpated with moderate fat covering. Waist poorly discernible. Obvious rounding of abdomen. Moderate abdominal fat pad.

8. Ribs not palpable with excess fat covering. Waist absent. Obvious rounding of abdomen with prominent abdominal fat pad. Fat deposits present over lumbar area.

9. Ribs not palpable under heavy fat cover. Heavy fat deposits over lumbar area, face and limbs. Distention of abdomen with no waist. Extensive abdominal fat deposits.

Bjornvad CR, et al. Evaluation of a nine-point body condition scoring system in physically inactive pet cats. AJVR 2011;72:433-437.
Laflamme DP. Development and validation of a body condition score system for cats. A clinical tool. Feline Pract 1997;25:13-18.

©2013. All rights reserved.

FIGURE 2.1 (*Continued from the previous page*)

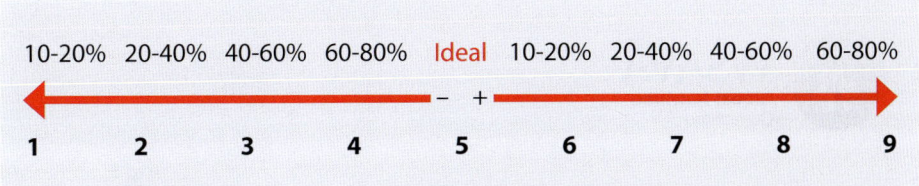

■ **FIGURE 2.2** Increase or decrease in percentage regarding to the ideal weight.

BOX 2.1 EXAMPLE OF THE CALCULATION OF THE IDEAL WEIGHT

Dog, weight 15 kg, BCS 7/9

20-40% overweight (3-6 kg)

Ideal weight: 9-12 kg

---

7. Ribs hardly palpable, adipose lining found often; appreciable fat deposits in the lumbar region and at the base of the tail; abdominal girdle absent or barely mentioned; mild abdominal retraction.
8. Ribs not palpable under a thick fatty coating or palpable only with significant pressure; thick deposits of fat in the lumbar region and at the base of the tail; abdominal girdle not distinguishable; abdominal retraction absent; noticeable abdominal distension.
9. Massive deposits of fat on the chest, spine and base of the tail; abdominal girdle not distinguishable; abdominal retraction absent; fat deposits on the neck and limbs; marked abdominal distension.

The MCS, on the other hand, evaluates – always through observation and palpation – the muscle mass. In this case, the parts to be evaluated are the thigh, the vertebrae, the temporal bones and the pelvic bones (Figure 2.3).

There are divided in four categories: normal, mild, moderate, severe. It is important to evaluate BCS and MCS together, especially in older animals suffering from different pathologies.

The third step is to choose the right food. Whether it is commercial, homemade, wet, dry, raw, etc., the important thing is that it is appreciated/consumed by the animal and that it meets the owner's expectations and needs.

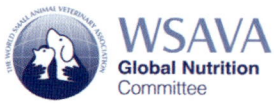

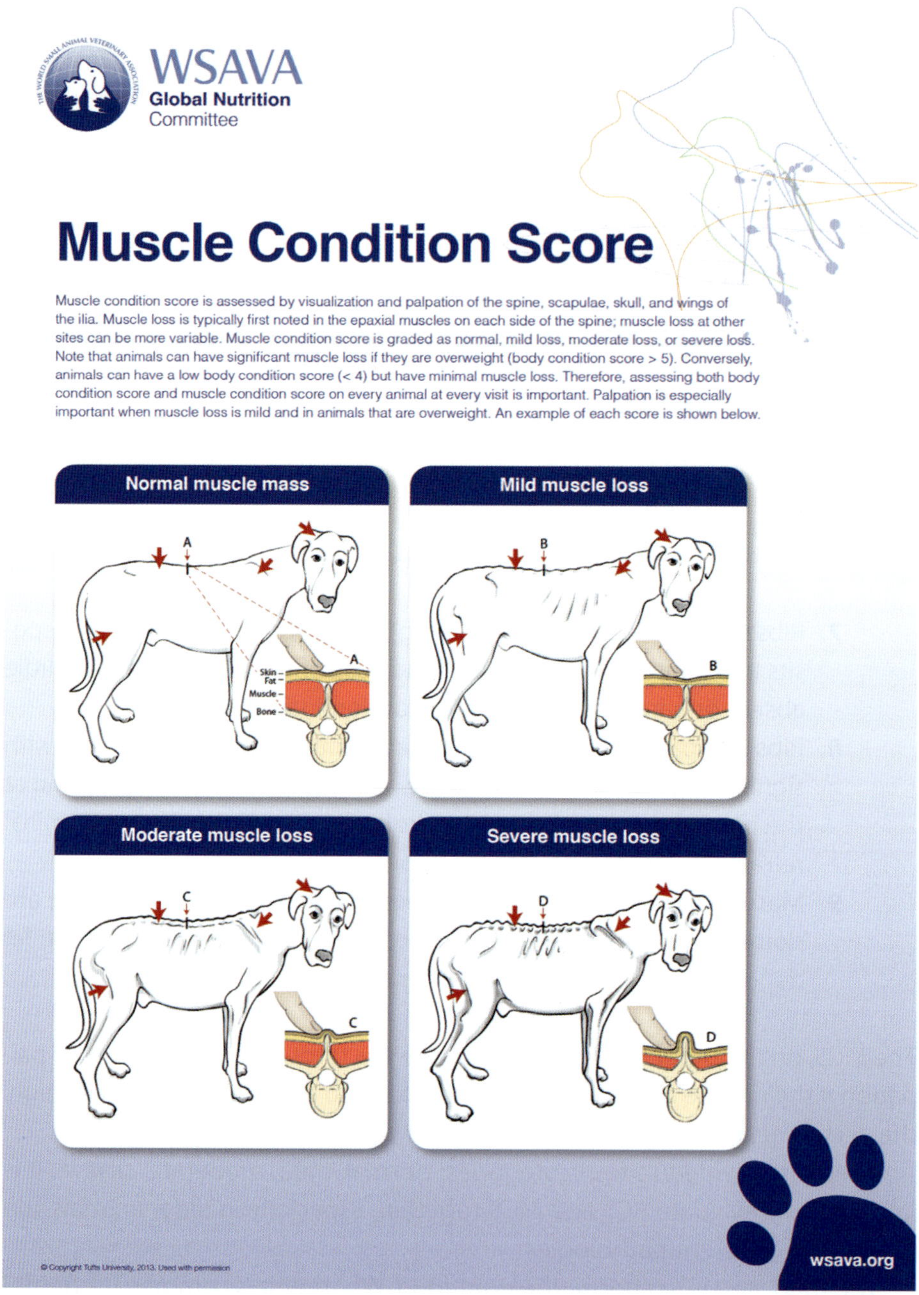
WSAVA
Global Nutrition
Committee
Muscle Condition Score
Muscle condition score is assessed by visualization and palpation of the spine, scapulae, skull, and wings of the ilia. Muscle loss is typically first noted in the epaxial muscles on each side of the spine; muscle loss at other sites can be more variable. Muscle condition score is graded as normal, mild loss, moderate loss, or severe loss. Note that animals can have significant muscle loss if they are overweight (body condition score > 5). Conversely, animals can have a low body condition score (< 4) but have minimal muscle loss. Therefore, assessing both body condition score and muscle condition score on every animal at every visit is important. Palpation is especially important when muscle loss is mild and in animals that are overweight. An example of each score is shown below.
Normal muscle mass
A
Skin
Fat
Muscle
Bone
Mild muscle loss
B
Moderate muscle loss
C
Severe muscle loss
D
© Copyright Tufts University, 2013. Used with permission
wsava.org

■ **FIGURE 2.3** Muscle Condition Score (MCS). *Provided courtesy of the World Small Animal Veterinary Association (WSAVA). Available at the WSAVA Global Nutrition Committee Nutritional Toolkit website: https://www.wsava.org/nutrition-toolkit. Accessed June 29, 2016. Copyright Tufts University, 2014.*

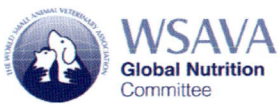

Muscle Condition Score

Muscle condition score is assessed by visualization and palpation of the spine, scapulae, skull, and wings of the ilia. Muscle loss is typically first noted in the epaxial muscles on each side of the spine; muscle loss at other sites can be more variable. Muscle condition score is graded as normal, mild loss, moderate loss, or severe loss. Note that animals can have significant muscle loss even if they are overweight (body condition score > 5/9). Conversely, animals can have a low body condition score (< 4/9) but have minimal muscle loss. Therefore, assessing both body condition score and muscle condition score on every animal at every visit is important. Palpation is especially important with mild muscle loss and in animals that are overweight. An example of each score is shown below.

Normal muscle mass	Mild muscle loss
Skin Fat Muscle Bone — Normal muscle mass — A	Mild muscle loss — B

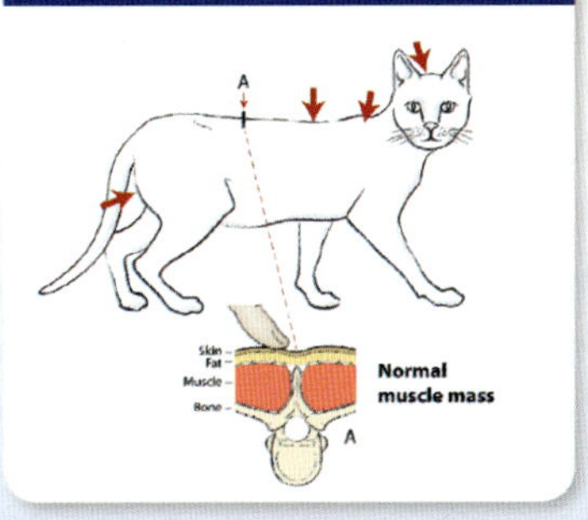

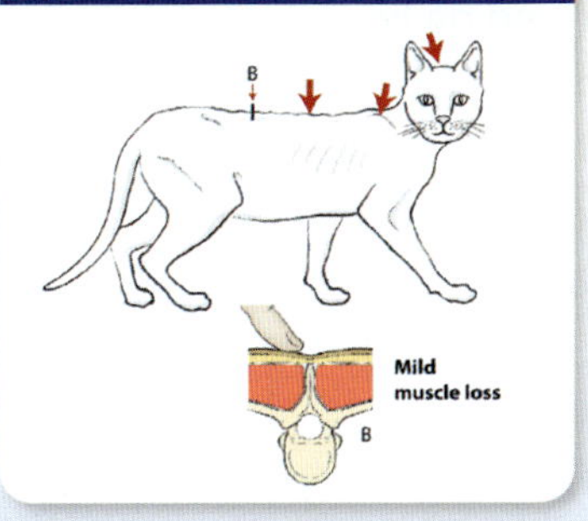

Moderate muscle loss	Severe muscle loss
Moderate muscle loss — C	Severe muscle loss — D

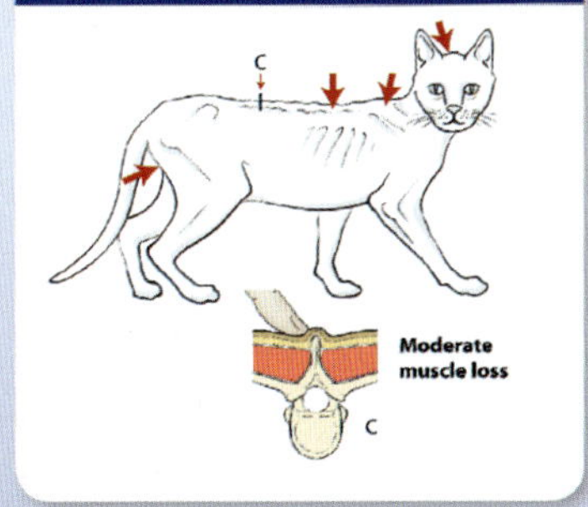

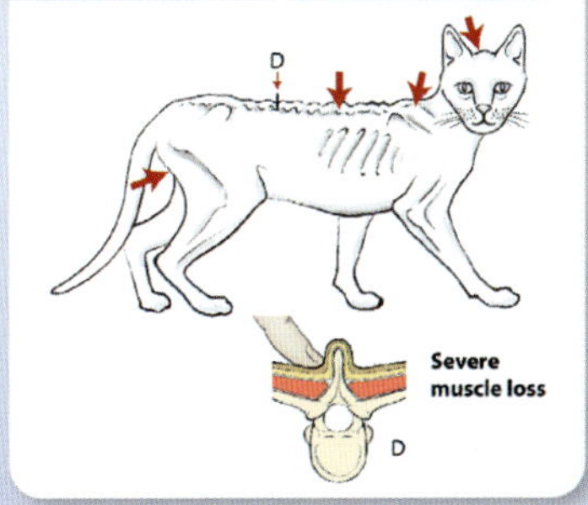

© Copyright Tufts University, 2014. Used with permission

wsava.org

Remember that the owner's compliance is fundamental. It is important that the owner understands the indications given to them, that they follow them carefully and, above all, this happens constantly.

In fact, we focus on the technical-scientific aspects very often leaving aside the emotional aspects. We should always explain to the owner why we choose that particular food for their animal and we must always ask them, by checking subsequently, if the animal eats willingly. In this way we will be able to maintain control over what the animal assumes and we will avoid the "do-it-yourself".

Last but not least, we must ration the meal: by calculating the kcal of the animal needs and those contained in the food. We must indicate the quantities to be administered daily.

Even if we have the reference tables shown on the packages and handbooks, it is advisable to redo the calculations by re-evaluating the dose and weight of the animal after at least a month, and in all cases, more often over time. It is advisable to always include any premiums in the total calculation of the daily kcal.

Obviously, all these elements must always be verified and re-evaluated over time (Figure 2.4).

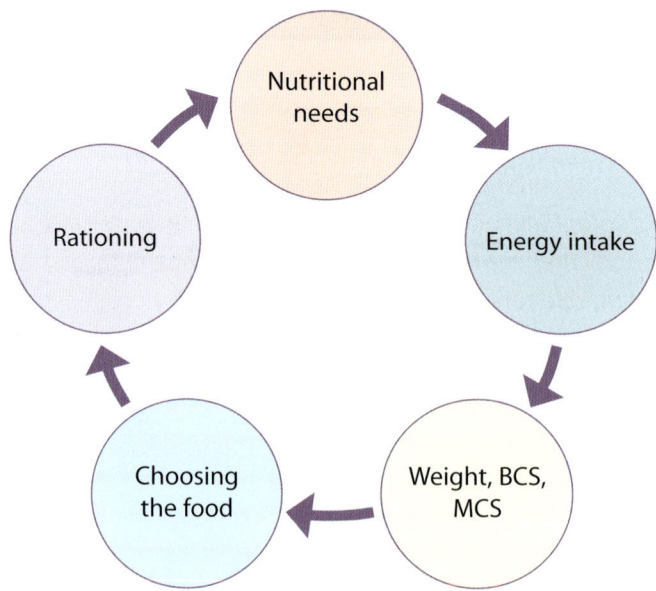

FIGURE 2.4 Elements to evaluate and re-evaluate over time.

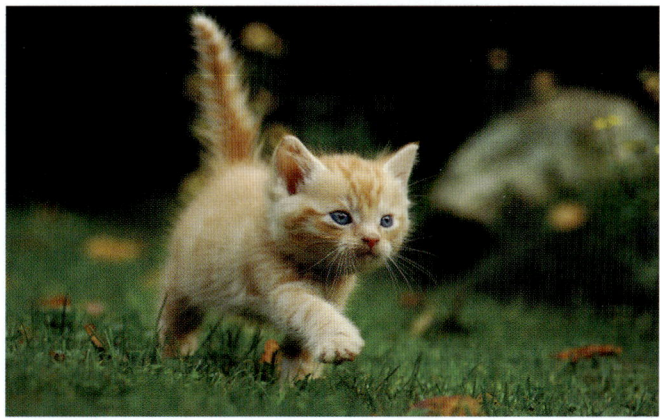

■ **FIGURE 2.5** A balanced diet is essential for the correct development of the kitten.

Puppies and kittens

A balanced diet during growth is a crucial factor for normal musculoskeletal development and for reducing the risks of viral, bacterial and parasitic infections (Figure 2.5). In this stage of animal life there is exceptional growth and development in a relatively short time. Large dogs reach normal adult size at 15-24 months of age. Small and medium sized dogs and cats at around 12 months of age.

Digestive and metabolic changes occur in the first 4-8 weeks of life in order to make puppies ready to start being introduced to foods other than milk and it is possible to start weaning.

4-6 week old kittens and 8 week old puppies are also able to chew dry food. In this period it is important to provide complete, energy and protein foods, but above all they must be extremely digestible. It is preferable to introduce one new ingredient at a time or monoproteinic foods especially during the first weaning period. The first 6 months of life represent the fastest growth phase, then the growth rate tends to slow down. The *energy needs* exceeds that of any other period of life, except for the breastfeeding period. The energy demands of puppies are about double of those of the adult. To calculate the kcal, the maintenance requirement must be multiplied by some correction factors related to the current weight. It is calculated as a percentage of the weight that the animal will have as an adult (Tables 2.1 and 2.2).

Obviously, for purebred dogs or in cases where the genealogy is known, the calculation will be simpler; for others, only assumptions and estimates can be made, and their growth followed.

■ **TABLE 2.1 - PUPPY'S CORRECTION FACTORS**

Puppy weight/Adult weight	Coefficient
30%	2.14
40%	1.94
50%	1.75
60%	1.58
70%	1.42
80%	1.28
90%	1.14

■ **TABLE 2.2 - KITTEN'S CORRECTION FACTORS**

Kitten's weight/Adult weight	Coefficient
<50% of the adult's weight	3
50-70% of the adult's weight	2.5
>70% of the adult's weight	2

Growth needs of the puppy

Multiplication coefficient of the maintenance requirement. For example: A puppy, 4 months old, weights 10 kg; adult weight hypothesized around 30 kg.

$$10 : 25 = x : 100$$

$$x = 40\%$$

Therefore, the coefficient to be used is 1.94. The maintenance requirement will then be calculated as follows:

$$10^{0.75} \times 110 = 618$$

and multiply it by the coefficient found:

$$kcal = 618 \times 1.94 = 1,198$$

Growth needs of the kitten

Multiplication coefficient of the maintenance requirement. For example: A kitten, 6 months old, weighs 2 kg, lives at home; adult weight 4-5 kg.

$$2 : 4 = x : 100$$

$$x = 50\%$$

Therefore, the coefficient to be used is 2.5. The maintenance requirement will then be calculated as follows:

$$2^{0.75} \times 70 = 117$$

and multiply it by the coefficient found:

$$kcal = 117 \times 2,5 = 292$$

 In this phase it is essential to avoid overeating, which can predispose the animal to obesity and skeletal pathologies. In the past, deficiency pathologies were common, but today we observe more frequently pathologies from excesses.

Proteins

The *protein requirement* is higher than that of an adult, since proteins are also used for the synthesis of new tissues. They must be of high quality and very digestible.

In growing dogs there are no studies that show, as for energy, the harmful effects from the excess protein intake, but remember that the digestive and renal capacity is lower under 8 weeks of life.

A protein deficiency can lead to reduction in growth, weight loss, less resistance to infections and alterations in brain development. Particular attention must be paid especially to kittens, in which over 60% of the ingested proteins are used for maintenance and only 40% for growth. As for puppies, these odds are 34 and 66% respectively (Figures 2.6 and 2.7).

For this reason, it is even more important that the protein intake is always adequate and monitored, especially in kittens.

The protein needs in puppies and kittens are different from the adult, not only quantitatively, but also qualitatively. At this stage, not only essential amino acids are important, but also non-essential ones. In kittens, *taurine deficiency* can lead to alterations of the retina and dilated myocardiopathy within 5-6 months. However, taurine seems more available in kittens, perhaps due to a lower degradation by bacteria in the intestine.

In puppies, however, if methionine and cystine are present in sufficient concentrations, the latter are able to synthesize it.

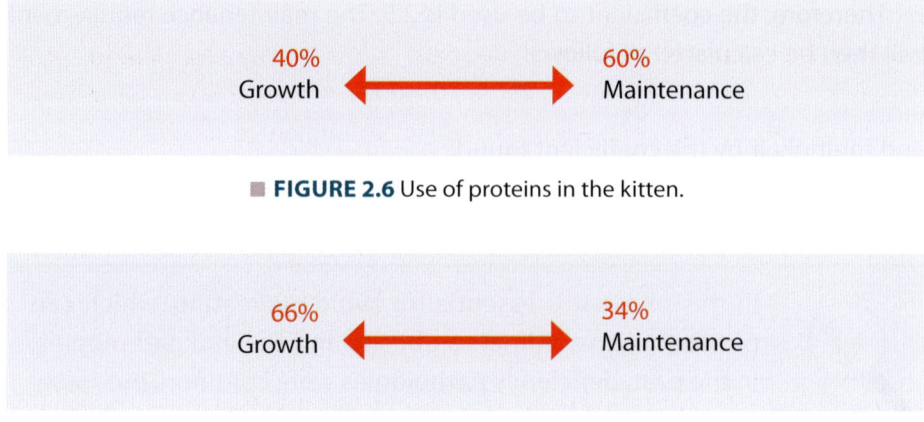

40%
Growth

60%
Maintenance

■ **FIGURE 2.6** Use of proteins in the kitten.

66%
Growth

34%
Maintenance

■ **FIGURE 2.7** Use of proteins in the puppy.

Amino acids

Arginine is an essential amino acid. Generally in adult cats and in kittens, but also in puppies, a deficiency of it, can lead to *hyperammonemia*. Arginine deficiency can also be relative when the protein level is high. It is estimated that for each 1% of extra protein on the dry matter (DM), arginine must be increased proportionally by 0.01 g in the dog and 0.02 g in the cat food. In puppies and kittens, a deficiency of arginine and histidine can also lead to the onset of *cataracts, anorexia, reduced growth*.

Non-essential amino acids such as *phenylalanine* and *tyrosine* are also important. Their deficiency can lead to alterations of protein metabolism, production of thyroid hormones and catecholamines, or even to a simple alteration of the coat color, especially if it is black.

Fats

Fats are essential for the animal, especially during their growth: they carry energy, essential fatty acids and fat-soluble vitamins. They are important for the skin, the hair, the development of the nervous system, the regulation of inflammation and the immune system etc. Among the fatty acids, one with a great interest is obviously linolenic acid (LA), but also omega-6 arachidonic acid (ARA), alfalinoleic acid (ALA), docosahexaenoic acid (DHA) omega-3, omega-3 eicosapentaenoic acid (EPA), which are essential in puppies, unlike the adults.

The lack of DHA and EPA leads to insufficient development of the nervous system, retina and auditory system. In puppies, the conversion of short chain fatty acids into DHA is not efficient, therefore the intake of DHA through the diet is considered essential during growth.

Minerals and vitamins

Minerals and vitamins are always important, but they play a fundamental role especially in puppies and kittens. It is necessary to optimize growth without incurring deficiencies, excesses or imbalances, which could determine the development of skeletal pathologies, and alterations of the immune and integumentary systems especially in large and giant dogs.

We have seen that *calcium deficiency* causes secondary hyperparathyroidism and excess calcitriol and, in severe cases, fractures, slowed growth rate, rickets etc. The calcium/phosphorus ratio is always important, but even more at this stage. We must be very careful, because puppies, in addition to the active absorption of calcium, also have passive absorption for the first 6 months of life. This preserves them from deficiencies, but puts them at risk of excess.

The *excess of calcium* causes alterations of the skeletal metabolism: an increase in the activity of osteoblasts, a decrease in the activity of osteoclasts and also an increase in bone mass and cartilaginous cones. This can lead to curved radius, osteochondrosis, enostosis etc.

Vitamin D is important because it increases the levels of calcium and phosphorus in the blood through the increase in renal and intestinal reabsorption. Vitamin D deficiency causes the same alterations as calcium deficiency does. However, even the excess is harmful and involves ectopic calcifications and severe intoxication in puppies and kittens, which can die even in a 2-5 week period.

Zinc deficiency causes skin changes, immune system dysfunction and growth reduction. In general, it is linked to unbalanced diets ("generic dry food disease") or diets which are too rich in calcium. Large and giant dogs are the most predisposed.

Many pet foods contain adequate amounts of *copper*, but sometimes this element is not available. In puppies with copper deficiency, there is a loss of coat pigmentation (graying or brown/black), hyperextension of the distal phalanges and frontal opening of the fingers, and signs of normochromic normocytic anemia.

The *potassium* in the kitten is very important and the demand is high. Deficiency can lead to post-weaning hypokalemic syndrome, which leads to reduced growth, depression and motor problems. It is often linked to a high level of protein in the diet or to the use, in this period of life, of acidifying diets.

Prebiotics, probiotics and nucleotides are always useful, especially in puppies. Prebiotics and probiotics have been mentioned in the previous chapter.

Nucleotides are considered semi-essential nutrients. They are the precursors of DNA and RNA and are composed of a sugar, a nitrogen base and of one to three phosphate groups. Depending on the base, they are classified into purines and pyrimidines. They promote the repair and defenses of the intestinal mucosa, protect against diarrhea and reduce recovery times, promote the growth of lactobacilli and bifidobacteria and increase the humoral and cellular immune capacity; they also have positive effects on liver regeneration. Many tissues such as bone marrow, liver, intestinal mucosa and immune cells have a capacity, even if it is limited, to produce them from scratch.

From a metabolic point of view, their production is difficult and "expensive", especially in young and immunocompromised animals.

Plant-based foods are poor in nucleotides, while animal-based foods have a certain number of them, but are scarcely available, especially for young and old animals. Breast milk is rich in nucleotides, except for cow's milk. For this reason, when it is necessary, its presence in foods or supplements must be verified.

📩☞ How many times a day do puppies and kittens have to eat?

During weaning, start with little and multiple meals, then continue with four to five times a day, with three main meals and two lighter meals for a dog; small and frequent meals are always recommended for cats.

The adult

The nutritional needs of the adult animal are influenced by weight, sterilization, environmental temperature and the animal's temperament. The administration of an adequate quantity of high quality and well formulated food will help to maintain the ideal body weight and an optimal state of health, preventing and slowing down the onset of diseases (Figure 2.8).

Unfortunately, at this stage of the animal's life, it is paid very little attention and only a few checks are performed.

Overweight and obesity are very frequent "diseases" at this stage of life, especially in sterilized animals. For this reason, it is important to monitor the weight of the animal and, if necessary, change the quantity or type of food taken.

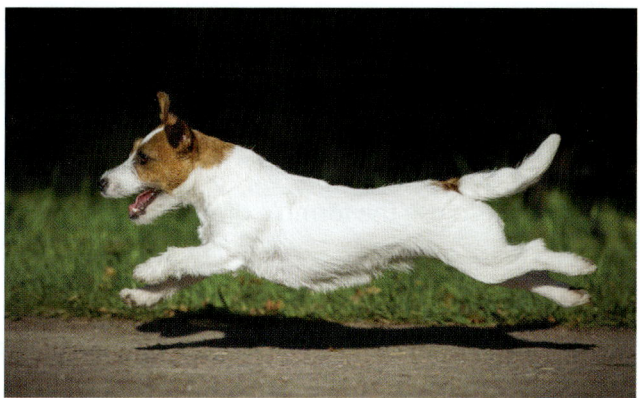

■ **FIGURE 2.8** To maintain optimal health of the adult dog, it is essential to provide them with high quality and properly formulated food.

For the same weight, a sterilized animal needs about 20-30% less energy than an unsterilized animal, therefore we must recommend a dedicated balanced food. In fact, you cannot simply reduce the doses of the food that was administered previously, without causing deficiencies and nutritional imbalances.

As we all know, overweight or obese animals have a higher risk of developing chronic diseases such as diabetes, lung and cardiovascular diseases, joint problems etc. Therefore, we must pay great attention to the type and quantity of food eaten, but also to treats and snacks.

A recent study reports that approximately 56.8% of dogs and 26.1% of cats receive treats/snacks. Based on our experience in dogs, it is over 90%. For various reasons, treats and snacks are an important element of the human-animal relationship, but we recommend planning them, avoiding the "do it yourself". Sometimes they cover up to 40% of the necessary kilocalories, while it is advisable that they should not exceed 10% of the daily requirement. Pay attention to treats such as dried meat, frankfurters or similar foods, which are obviously highly appreciated by animals, because they significantly increase the daily protein intake, unbalancing the diet. It is useless to ban treats and snacks, but one must learn to limit them and calculate them in the diet of the animals.

👉 How should the maintenance needs of a sterilized/neutered dog or cat be calculated?

The maintenance requirement must be calculated with the formulas seen above and must be multiplied by a correction factor of 0.8 (Table 2.3)

■ TABLE 2.3 - CALCULATION OF THE ENERGY REQUIREMENT OF A STERILIZED/ NEUTERED ANIMAL

Maintenance needs	Multiplication factor
MN = 110 x (weight in kg)$^{0.75}$	0.8

For the cat you can also use the formula directly:

$$MN = 60 \times \text{weight in kg}$$

■☛ How many times a day do sterilized/neutered dogs and cats eat?

At least twice a day for dogs, 3-4 times or even more for the cat (it is always better to divide it into little and frequent meals). It is not necessary to offer a wide variety of foods. A constant diet, which prevents gastrointestinal complaints such as vomiting and diarrhea, is more appropriate.

Aging

Nutrition plays a fundamental role in the control of aging, preventing or slowing down the onset of diseases associated with age and improving symptoms, quality of life and therefore the life span (Figure 2.9). At this stage of life there is a natural decrease in physical activity and a change in body composition, in fat tissues which is in favor of lean tissues. This implies a *reduction of the daily requirement of even 30-40%* (Figure 2.10). In the first phase, the energy intake will therefore have to decrease, to avoid diseases such as obesity or dia-

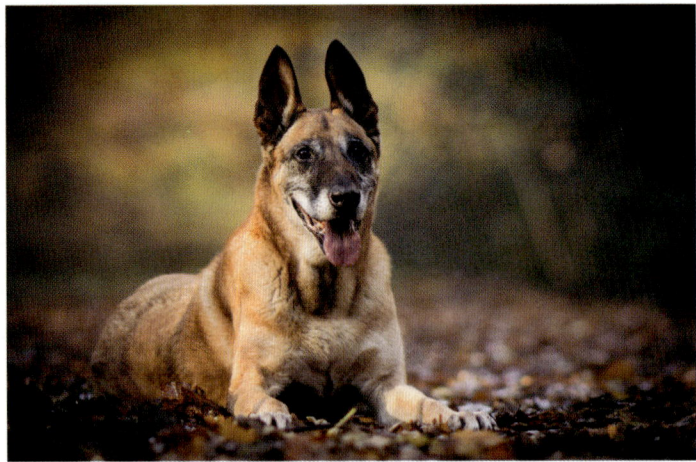

■ FIGURE 2.9 In an elderly dog, proper nutrition plays an essential role in the prevention of the diseases.

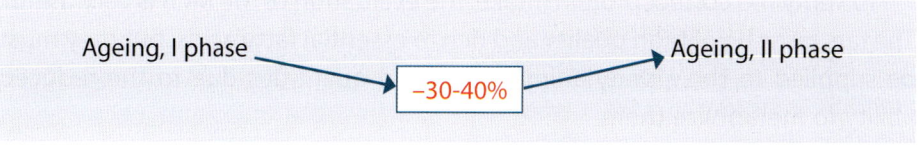

Ageing, I phase

−30-40%

Ageing, II phase

FIGURE 2.10 The course of energy needs in the elderly.

betes mellitus, but then it will have to increase again and it will be necessary to counteract the loss of lean mass which is typical of the elderly. In cats, this occurs mostly around the age of 13, but there is a certain variability and the individual subject must be evaluated.

 The evaluation of BCS and MCS is always important, but in elderly animals it becomes fundamental, especially for the physiological changes in the relationship between lean mass and fat mass.

In elderly animals, cell and tissue renewal rate also decreases, the skin loses elasticity and they can have hyperkeratosis, the appearance of alopecic areas and loss of pigment of the follicles, with the appearance of white hair especially on the muzzle. The ability to eliminate catabolites, especially proteins, is reduced and chronic diseases such as kidney failure are often present, which represents one of the most frequent chronic diseases in dogs and it holds the first place in cats. It decreases the ability to ingest, digest and metabolize food.

Age predisposes some elderly animals also to constipation, because of the reduction of colon motility.

Unfortunately, the reference values for this phase of life are not reported in the FEDIAF tables, therefore it is essential to evaluate the general state of health of the animal and gradually adapt the feeding based on the changes that occur over time, to the needs of the moment or the onset of any pathologies.

Proteins must be supplied in adequate quantities, they should be of high biological value and extremely digestible. For some years, a mistake that was made was to decrease them in order to prevent kidney problems: in Chapter 4 it will be indicated if and when it is appropriate to do so. It must always be kept in mind that it has been shown that the elderly dog has a protein requirement of at least 20% of the dry substance, while in the cat this requirement is even higher, because this animal remains a "super carnivore" at any age.

To verify the correct protein intake, the evaluation of the MCS is very useful. The fats must be of high quality and rich in essential fatty acids, but they must be supplied to the elderly animal in limited quantities due to the reduced ability to metabolize them.

Immune defenses and the body's ability to eliminate free radicals also decreases, so it is essential to provide, especially in this period, antioxidant substances and vitamins, such as *vitamin E*. Among the vitamins in general, those that are the most important are B-group vitamins, which are necessary for the use of carbohydrates due to the reduced glucose tolerance, typical for this age. In fact, it is important to reduce the glycemic index of the ration to try to prevent diseases such as diabetes mellitus, possibly also using dedicated carbohydrates such as barley and sorghum. However, frequent checks are recommended, at least once every 4-6 months.

☞ How many times a day should elderly animals eat?

We must consider the elderly as "special puppies": they should eat little and frequently. Especially at this stage of life, abrupt changes in feeding should be avoided.

Pregnancy

Feeding and caring for pregnant animals are essential for their health and fitness and for the vitality, health and growth of puppies (Figure 2.11). Proper nutrition should ideally begin during the growth and development of the parents and continue during mating, pregnancy and breastfeeding. It is very important that especially the female, is in optimal physical condition before mating.

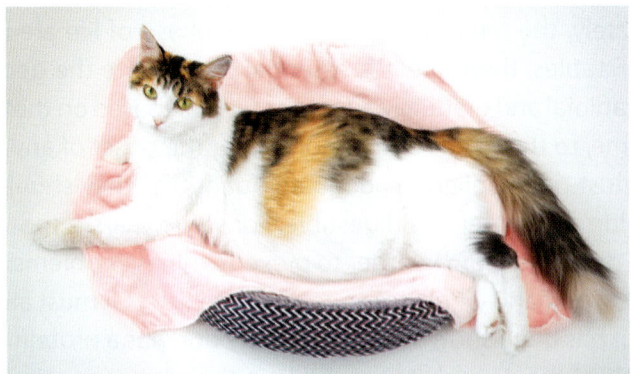

■ **FIGURE 2.11** In order for the pregnancy to continue in optimal mode, the cat's feeding must be particularly cared for.

If the animal is underweight, or even overweight, its fertility is significantly reduced, with a decrease in the number of offspring, silent heats, difficulty in childbirth and greater neonatal mortality. A pregnant dog and cat should be fed with a high quality, highly digestible, energy food.

Contrary to the popular belief, it is not necessary to change the type of food or increase its quantity immediately after fecundation. It should be done gradually after the 4th-5th week in dogs (last third of the pregnancy) and after the second week in cats, to avoid excessive weight gain and, therefore, any problems, especially at birth (Figures 2.12 and 2.13).

The energy requirement of a pregnant dog increases on average by 30-60% compared to that of maintenance, also as a function of the number of fetuses; in cats it increases by 25-50% and is independent of the number of fetuses (Table 2.4).

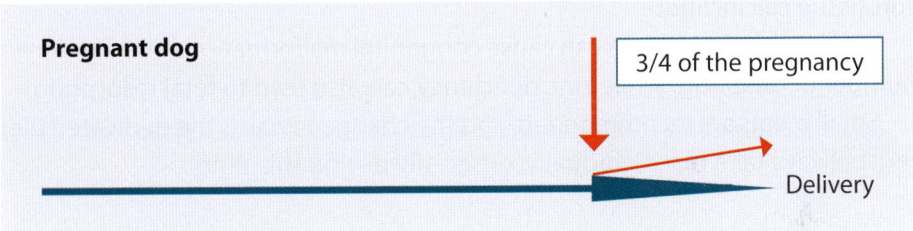

■ **FIGURE 2.12** Increased kcal after three quarters of the pregnancy.

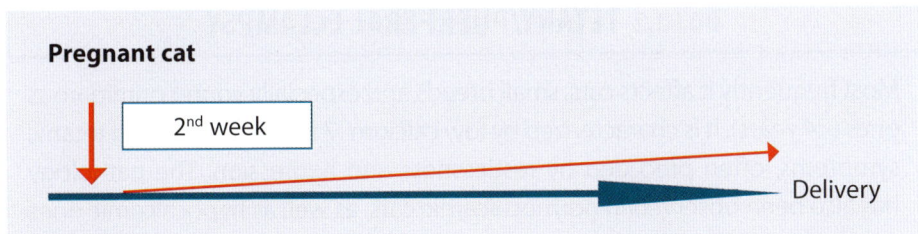

■ **FIGURE 2.13** Gradual increase in kcal throughout the period of pregnancy, starting from the second week.

■ **TABLE 2.4 - CALCULATION OF THE ENERGY REQUIREMENT IN PREGNANCY IN DOGS AND IN CATS**

Gestation	Maintenance energy	× 1.25-1.5

In this phase, we must pay great attention to the proteins and amino acids such as arginine, methionine, tryptophan and, always to taurine in cats. Not only are the quantities of proteins very important, but also their composition and digestibility. Attention should also be paid to fats, in particular to some fatty acids already treated previously, such as linoleic acid, alpha-linolenic acid, arachidonic acid, EPA and DHA.

Unlike before, during this period we must pay attention to the carbohydrates (>23% DM). More than 50% of the energy for fetal development is provided by glucose, therefore at least 10-20% of the energy supplied by the food should derive from carbohydrates. For this reason, the most important of the vitamins is thiamine (vitamin B_1), which has a fundamental role in regulating carbohydrate metabolism.

It is very important to maintain the correct mineral and vitamin levels. deficiencies are dangerous, as are the excesses. The correct levels of calcium and phosphorus are fundamental. Their deficiency, for example, can lead to uterine inertia, impaired ossification of fetuses and skeletal problems in puppies.

An excess of calcium and/or vitamin D can cause eclampsia (Box 2.2) and soft tissue calcification.

The excess of vitamin A can cause congenital malformations and a reduced number of offspring, while zinc deficiency can also lead to fetal resorption.

Small meals are recommended, and the change towards the dedicated diet must always take place gradually, especially during this time.

BOX 2.2 TETANY/PUERPERAL ECLAMPSY

Most frequently it affects cats, small breeds and especially young primiparous ones (<4 years). It is characterized by low calcium (7 mg/dL or less) and tetanic symptoms, often preceded by restlessness and aggression. The pathology has also been observed in normocalcemic cats, as well as hypocalcemic ones which may have no symptoms. It must be treated promptly and the puppies must be separated from the mother during the first 24 hours of therapy. If it is repeated, a definitive separation should be made. It is important to avoid excess calcium during pregnancy (negative feedback effect on the parathyroid hormone) and to ensure an adequate intake after delivery, to compensate for the strong losses due to lactation.

Feeding time

Breastfeeding represents one of the biggest nutritional challenges, since in this period the energy and various nutrient needs are increased even more, reaching the maximum peak during the fourth week after giving birth in dogs and the seventh week in cats (Figure 2.14).

The food must be of high quality, digestible and high in energy. In the FEDIAF tables you can find references regarding the needs of proteins, fats, vitamins and minerals, which are in fact superimposable to the first phase of growth (<14 weeks) in dogs and in general growth in cats. In this phase, the animal needs to consume three to four times more energy which is needed for maintenance. Obviously, this will also depend to a considerable extent on the number of puppies present (Table 2.5).

Even in lactation, 10-20% of the metabolizable energy must come from carbohydrates. Water is always essential, but in this period an insufficient water supply leads to a considerable reduction in the quantity of produced milk (Figure 2.15). Generally, towards the 4th-6th week after giving birth in cats and the 7th-8th week in dogs, begins the weaning of the kittens/puppies. During this period, the mother's food consumption should not exceed 50% of the maintenance consumption (as in the end of pregnancy), so it will be important to start decreasing it gradually in the previous weeks.

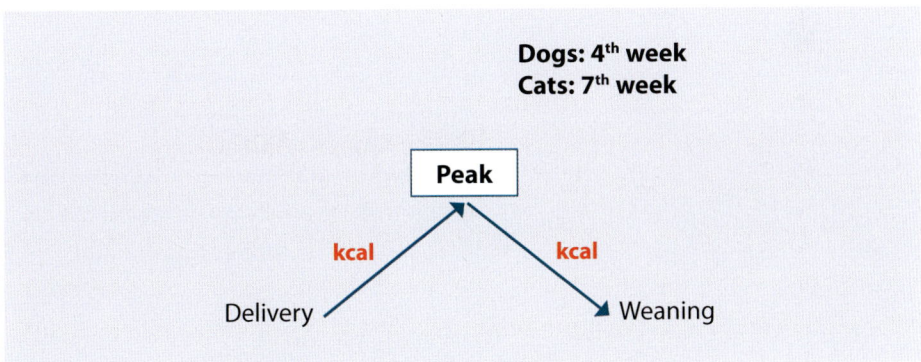

FIGURE 2.14 Trends in lactation energy needs.

TABLE 2.5 - CALCULATION OF THE ENERGY REQUIREMENT DURING LACTATION IN DOGS AND CATS

Feeding time	Maintenance energy	× 3-4

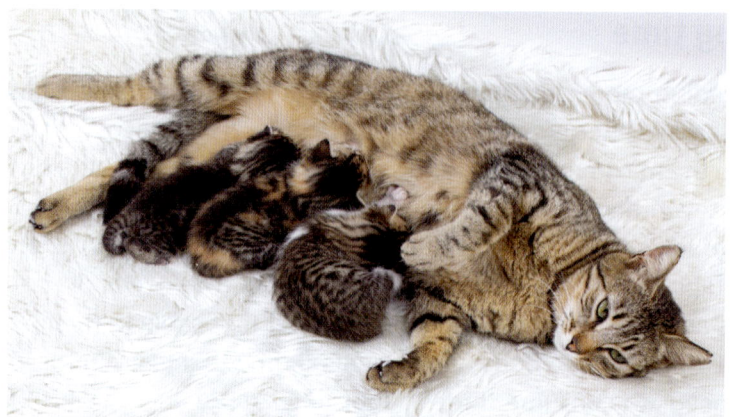

■ **FIGURE 2.15** During breastfeeding, it is particularly important to make sure that the cat takes the correct amount of water.

In general, during breastfeeding, the animals undergo natural weight loss, however it must not exceed 10% of the normal body weight. If feeding and care during pregnancy and breastfeeding have been adequate, the mother's weight loss is reduced to a minimum and even for large offspring, her recovery will be faster and the puppies will be viable and in optimal condition.

It is better to provide small and frequent meals during the day, to avoid exceeding the digestive capacity. An *ad libitum* diet can also be recommended, so that the animals can self-regulate.

Chapter 3

The foods

Commercial or fresh, the important thing
is that it is complete, balanced and ... eaten

OBJECTIVES OF THIS CHAPTER
• Knowing the various types of foods • Knowing how to read a label

Today we have a large number of foods available, natural or commercial, which differ in the type of cooking, the percentage of water, the type of ingredients, etc.

What to recommend? Which one to choose? We will see the pros and cons of the different types, we will understand how to evaluate commercial foods by reading the label and we will find out what are the most important characteristics that can and must guide us.

Choosing the food

There are essentially three characteristics that we must keep in mind when we choose a food: nutritional adequacy, palatability, digestibility. However, in our opinion, there is also a fourth characteristic, the owner (Figure 3.1).

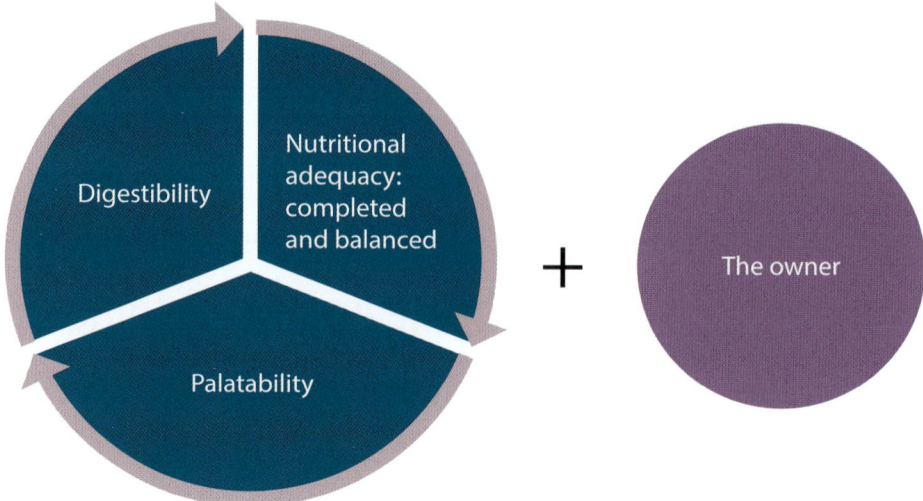

■ **FIGURE 3.1** The four characteristics on the basis of which we choose a food.

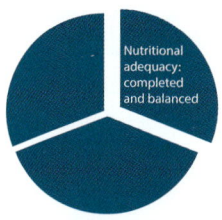
First of all, as we have seen in the previous chapters, the food must be complete and balanced, it must satisfy the caloric requirement and, at the same time, it must cover the requirement of all nutrients.

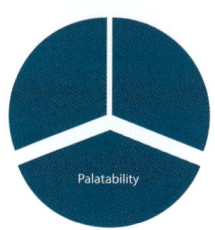
The food should also be palatable for the animal and this characteristic must be checked constantly over time, without resorting to "do it yourself". Contrary to popular belief, animals are unable to regulate the supply of nutrients. They eat to meet their energy needs: for this reason, our role is fundamental, if we want to avoid deficiencies or excesses.

We must explain to our customers that there is a big difference between palatability and nutritional adequacy and that they must not allow themselves to be influenced by the choices of the animal but follow our advice, since the animal does not choose the best or the best balanced food. We must always verify that the advice is accepted and followed over time, and possibly re-evaluate it if necessary (animals are not all the same).

When choosing, we must pay particular attention to cats. In nature, this animal hunts a large number of prey, making many attacks per day, of which only a small percentage is successful.

In addition, it catches different prey every time, which ensures its variability and nutritional adequacy. This could explain why cats that live in the house like to eat little and frequent meals, and also change the food often.

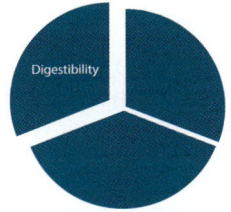

The digestibility of a food is also important, as it is closely linked both to the percentage of nutrients actually absorbed, therefore available, and to the general well-being of the animal. Food that is not digestible or poorly digested can lead to excessive fermentation, with gas production and it can increase intestinal peristalsis that results in poorly formed stools or even in diarrhea.

A digestible food, on the other hand, produces a reduced volume of stool, shaped and compact, without mucus or blood. The frequency of evacuation is not excessive (1-2 times a day) and bowel movements are regular and constant. We have available comparison tables that can help us interpret the feces (Faecal Scoring System). It is therefore important to always ask the owner for this information, possibly showing the comparison table if you have any doubts. Over time, we can and must reconsider the choice of food through the evaluation of the skin and coat, the maintenance of body weight, regular growth etc.

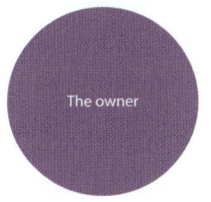

Last but not least, although it may seem strange, the choice of food also depends, as already mentioned above, on the owner, their expectations, the times they are available, their predisposition or their beliefs. Keep this in mind: it allows you to have more control over the food consummation and to avoid "do it yourself".

Pre-packaged foods (commercial)

Prepackaged foods, according to the water content and the method of conservation and the processing, can be divided into dry and wet. Dry foods contain 6-10% water (moisture). Among these we can mention both biscuits and extrusions (croquettes). In biscuits, the ingredients are mixed in a dough which is then cut (modeled) and baked in the oven. The crunchies are produced in a machine called an extruder, which combines the action of the temperature with that of the pressure. The extrusion process improves the digestibility of complex carbohydrates (starches) and sterilizes the product.

Dry foods, in general, are cheaper than both wet and homemade food and are more easily preserved thanks to the low water content; they are certainly practical, complete and balanced, but are usually less palatable, therefore they are added with appetizing substances called "digest".

In general, dry foods are cheaper than both wet and homemade food and are more easily preserved thanks to the low water content; they are certainly practical, complete and balanced, but they are usually less palatable. Therefore, appetizing substances called "digest" are added to these foods.

Wet foods have a water content of around 75% and are prepared by cooking and mixing the ingredients, canning and then completing the cooking of the sealed container, which is thus sterilized. There are two types: complete and balanced ones, integrated with vitamins and minerals, and complementary ones, mainly made up of meat or fish alone. Wet foods are more palatable and digestible than the dry ones.

They are also practical but, once the container is opened, they must be consumed within a maximum of 48 hours; additionally, they have higher costs, especially for medium and large dogs. For cats, they would be preferable and / or possibly associated with dry ones. Nowadays, most owners use ready-made commercial foods, as they are on average cheaper (especially for medium-large dogs), easier to maintain, more complete and balanced, and above all they are faster to administer.

 Cats concentrate their urine a lot, so eating only dry foods could predispose them to lower urinary tract diseases such as cystitis and stones. On the other hand, dry foods are best suited to be used for their small and frequent meals.

Homemade food

 Homemade food is certainly more palatable than pre-packaged food, it undergoes fewer transformations, allows you to see and choose the ingredients, it can be of higher quality and digestibility. Several owners are oriented towards this type of diet for many reasons and the most frequent of which are: poor palatability of commercial foods, lack of trust in commercial food or, simply, the pleasure and desire to cook for their pet. The homemade diet can be done and above all it can be recommended. From a nutritional point of view, it is as reliable as the ones of good commercial quality, also for puppies. On the other hand, the

owner must have available time, a correctly formulated, balanced and integrated recipe, and must be able to rigorously respect the dosages and ingredients.

Recipe ingredients, as well as supplements, should never be replaced or eliminated. Checks are always important, but in this case they are even more important and it is necessary to verify that the diet has not undergone any changes and variations (drifts) over time.

Vegetarian and vegan diets

As explained above, dogs and cats are carnivores and a vegetarian or vegan diet is obviously a strain. Today, there are just a few studies on this topic and above all, they are limited in time. Cats, unless they take supplements, cannot be fed neither a vegetarian diet nor a vegan one. In fact, we have already seen how this animal needs different nutrients which are present exclusively in meat, fish, eggs, milk, animal fats etc.

Instead, it seems possible to feed dogs with a vegetarian diet, but not with a pure vegan one. We must remember that vegetable proteins are less digestible than animal proteins and, moreover, they contain phytates that can bind different minerals causing a deficiency (calcium, iron, zinc etc.). They may also contain protease inhibitors, hemagglutinins etc.

The critical factors that should be kept under control are essential amino acids, especially tryptophan, methionine and lysine, vitamin B_{12}, vitamin A and vitamin D. Nowadays, sometimes, vegetarian diets are given to dogs and have proven to be useful for animals which are intolerant or allergic to animal proteins. In any case, it is more appropriate to use commercial pre-packaged diets, which can better guarantee the presence of all essential nutrients; however, this is not obvious, so you have to be very careful and make frequent visits and checks.

The first BARF type diets

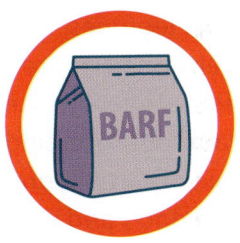

The continuous research for healthier and more natural diets has led to a huge development and use of BARF type diets, which follow the predator-prey concept. There are different conceptions and philosophies in the "correct raw" nutrition, of which the best known is the one called BARF, an abbreviation usually used with the meaning of Biologically Appropriate Raw Food.

They are characterized by raw meat, with a high percentage of bone, with pulp and internal organs (spleen, liver, lungs, intestine etc.). They also include raw vegetables and fruits, nuts, oils, herbs, algae, eggs and dairy products. They are almost free of carbohydrates, especially cereals. Raw meat is more digestible than cooked meat, but its use involves hygienic risks such as bacterial (*Escherichia coli*, *Salmonella*, *Campylobacter* and *Yersinia*) and parasitic (*Echinococcus*, *Toxoplasma* etc.) contaminations.

Parasitic contamination can be controlled by using frozen meat for at least 48 hours, but freezing does not prevent bacterial contamination. In this regard, we recommend, if necessary, the use of beef, which is subject to greater and more accurate health checks and is less contaminated on average; in fact, it is the only meat that can also be eaten raw by humans. Bones improve chewing and cleaning of teeth, but can cause various degrees of irritation and injury; moreover, it is difficult to control and balance the calcium, phosphorus and other minerals taken through their consumption.

It is also important to know that some ingredients are not suitable to be eaten raw, such as eggs, which contain avidin which binds to biotin (vitamin B_7) causing its deficiency; moreover, they contain a trypsin inhibitor which hinders the digestion of proteins.

Many raw fish contain thiaminase, which destroys thiamine (vitamin B_1), and may contain trimethylamine, which binds iron and can cause anemia.

These diets, with the necessary modifications, integrated and adequately balanced, can be a valid alternative to other diets, especially in some animals with gastrointestinal problems.

Grain-free and/or gluten-free diets

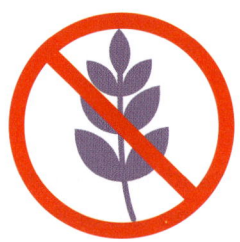

Grain-free diets are rich in proteins and free from cereals or gluten. They don't always have a low carbohydrate content, contrary to what many people think; indeed, these are simply present in different forms such as potatoes, peas, tapioca, legumes. Carbohydrates, especially cereals, have always been used and included in home and commercial diets, since they allow savings in the use of proteins and are important for processing and technological production processes. However, the role of carbohydrates – especially cereals – has come under scrutiny in both dog's and cat's diets. Today, on the market, there are numerous "Grain-free" or "gluten-free"

products that are enjoying great success and promise to improve and safeguard the health of the animal. However, unless an animal has a certain documented allergy to a cereal (which is quite rare), providing a diet without cereals or gluten does not bring any benefits.

There is also evidence that carbohydrates are not a direct risk factor for the development of diabetes in cats and dogs, and many studies have shown that carbohydrates are not associated with obesity, which rather seems linked to *ad libitum* nutrition and the high density of the diet (high fat content, which is paradoxically much higher in diets with low carbohydrate content).

However, it is true that the natural diet of dogs, and above all, the diet of cats, is low in carbohydrates and rich in proteins. Cats do not have salivary amylase and they have lower amounts of pancreatic amylase than dogs, but they are able to digest, assimilate and use carbohydrates, especially when they are treated and cooked. This is even more true for dogs, which are considered opportunistic carnivores. Dogs, unlike cats, but above all their cousin, the wolf, in the course of evolution and domestication, has developed the ability to digest carbohydrates (starches) better.

Currently there are no published studies that have examined the long-term differences between animals which are fed with "new diets" (raw diets, "grain-free", "gluten-free") and those fed with "old diets" (croquettes, tins), with the exception of studies on the digestibility of raw BARF diets. Today we do not have data that allow us to indicate the most appropriate diet and even to ascertain whether cereals can cause problems, or more problems, than other carbohydrates, in healthy animals. This, however, does not exclude the possibility of using these diets especially in animals that have shown improvements with their intake.

The "hypoallergenic" diets

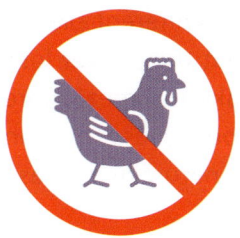

The term "hypoallergenic" is not exactly correct: in reality there is no hypoallergenic meat or food. A food may be hypoallergenic for one animal but may not be hypoallergenic for another. In general, hypoallergenic foods must be simple foods, with two or at most three ingredients, and contain new proteins and carbohydrate sources, that are never that have never been taken by the animal.

Paradoxically, chicken meat can be hypoallergenic for an animal that has never eaten it, despite being frequently identified as allergenic in many animals.

Several ingredients have been identified, that occur most frequently in allergies/adverse reactions to food, such as cattle, chicken, fish, dairy products etc. The diets recommended in the literature, especially in the diagnosis phase, are those which are prepared at home, as they guarantee a better control over the ingredients. If it is not possible to adopt them, commercial hydrolyzed diets can be used, but we do not recommend monoproteins since several studies have highlighted the presence of contaminations, which can be as much as 80% in dry diets and 20% in wet ones, affecting the results.

How and how often to feed your pet

This topic is very important, since we often pay close attention to which meal to give to our pet but we do not pay attention to the way we feed them, while it is also essential for its health and for a better coexistence.

The answers are given by taking into account the physiology, characteristics and the habits of our four-legged friends.

Dogs are a social animal and, for them, food also takes on a social role. It is recommended to feed a dog 2-3 times a day, as we have discussed previously. Furthermore, food should be left at its disposal only for a certain period of time, both for reasons related to the digestion and for behavioral reasons. Only one meal a day is not recommended, as it predisposes the dog to gastrointestinal pathologies, bad digestion and poor assimilation of nutrients.

The cat is a solitary animal, it eats very little and frequently, and gets stressed very easily. If there are multiple individuals, it is important that each one has their own bowl and raised and secluded places should be provided. Cats eat 15 times a day and, as we have seen, this protects it from certain pathologies. If possible, we must provide an *ad libitum* diet, possibly dividing the total meal of the day into several bowls positioned in different places. We must keep in mind that the cats are predator and that they never lose their hunting instinct, so we can use this instinct to make the meal more complicated, using prepared games or creating them ourselves. This can be very useful especially for overweight cats, in order to naturally increase their activity.

Snacks

It is advisable to use chewable snacks for playing or for training. There are found different types and shapes on the market (Figure 3.2) and today you can also find snacks completely made of vegetable, which are very useful for older animals that tend to gain weight, or for intolerant / allergic ones. Snacks are important for oral hygiene and for chewing in general, which strengthens the periodontium and controls stress. The ones we recommend most are pig ears, deer horns or simply dry bread. On the other hand, buffalo skin, bones and all snacks if excessively caloric, are absolutely to be avoided.

Dogs have the instinct to look for food and strive to obtain it: for this reason, food and snacks can be used for training or simply to let them play. However, we must pay attention to the calories that are provided by the various snacks. As we have seen above, they often represent a significant share of the kcal taken, while they should not exceed 10% of the daily total. So, we can use fruit (apple), vegetables (carrots), dry bread, commercial dry biscuits (simple), parmesan, cooked meat (grilled). We should also try to avoid commercial dehydrated meat or fish, raw frankfurters, raw meat.

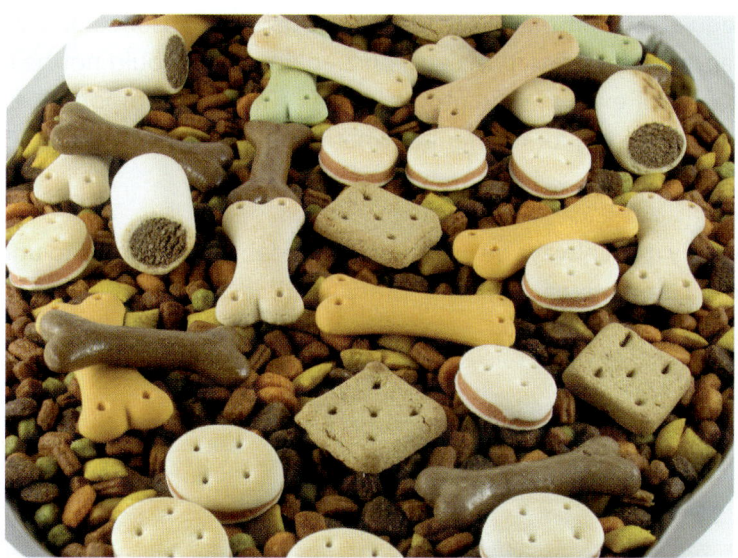

■ **FIGURE 3.2** Some examples of snacks available on the market, of different shapes, types and colors.

Even though snacks are not necessary for cats, they can be used to interact with them. However, it is important that they do not become the only form of contact with the pet. You can use pieces of grilled meat or croquettes that you do not use regularly. You can also use different croquettes, other than the regular ones.

Read the label

The information we can and must obtain from the label is different. Some can help us choose the most suitable food, others can serve to compare different products, but we must keep in mind that, by reading the label, we cannot truly evaluate the quality of a food and, above all, we cannot know its most important characteristic, digestibility, which is not among the information that must be reported. For this reason, the real judge of a food is only the animal.

The regulations regarding labels are different; the one with the greatest interest in Europe is Regulation (European Community, EC) 767/2009 which governs the conditions for placing food on the market and guarantees safety and adequate information to the consumer. In particular, this regulation aims to ensure that the information on the labels is clear and not misleading. Establishing this must be mandatory (type, species, composition, additives, etc.). It also regulates what may be optional (presence or absence of a substance, particular nutritional functions etc.) and, again, what should not be reported.

Here we will examine the indications that are most important in Europe (Figure 3.3), referring for further information to Regulation (EC) 767/2009.

Typology

The typology must always be indicated on the label. It allows us to understand if a food is complete or complementary and it is one of the first pieces of in-

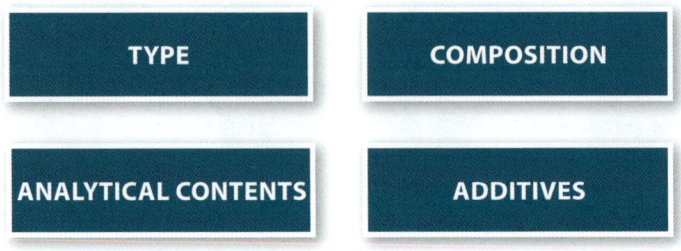

FIGURE 3.3 Important factors to evaluate on a label.

formation we need to look at when we choose a food. What is the difference between a complete and a complementary food? A complete food contains proteins, fats, generally also carbohydrates, and is integrated with vitamins and minerals; it can be given on its own and ensures that the animal has all the nutrients it needs.

A complementary food, on the other hand, mostly contains only one or a few ingredients, mostly protein sources, and is not integrated, therefore it must necessarily be given together with a balanced food or it must be integrated.

Wet foods are more often part of the complementary food category. The treatments the raw materials undergo (heat, grinding, dehydration etc.) lead to huge losses, especially of vitamins; moreover, a single ingredient obviously cannot ensure the presence of all the necessary nutrients. The use of only complementary foods can cause deficiencies, sometimes serious ones (Figure 3.4).

The composition

The composition is the list of the ingredients, which can be listed by name, such as chicken, beef, corn, rice etc. (open formula), or by category, such as meat and derivatives, cereals etc. (closed formula). The ingredients must be arranged according to their decreasing weight, from the most represented to the least represented.

The open formula allows us to know exactly which raw materials are used, but if we are not careful, we may lose the ingredient (or ingredients) that is most represented. The open formula involves the separation of the ingredients, even those belonging to the same category, which would otherwise be listed

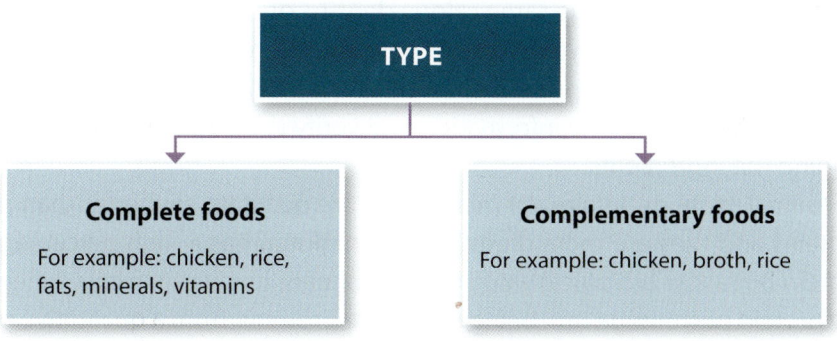

■ **FIGURE 3.4** Examples of the content of complete and complementary foods.

together and would end up in the recipe as the first ingredients. In the following example (open formula) meat is the main ingredient: chicken, corn, chicken fat, rice, carrots etc. With the closed formula the same example would become: cereals (corn + rice), meat, fats, vegetables etc., and meat would be listed as a second ingredient. So, to have meat as a main ingredient, just use different carbohydrate sources.

We must prefer products with an open formula and animal protein sources in the main ingredients and we must always read all the ingredients listed on the label, because this allows us to understand the actual representation of each individual ingredient.

Analytical contents

The analytical contents are the list of percentages of proteins, fats, fiber and ash that are mandatory to declare. Moisture should be declared only if it is higher than 14%, therefore only in wet foods. We must be careful, because they are expressed as such. For this reason, it is necessary that if we want to make comparisons, we should refer to the dry substance. In the case of dry foods such as croquettes, which have 8-10% moisture, this would not be a big problem but it is impossible to compare a dry food with a wet one, which has 60-80% moisture. We can therefore compare two foods only if they have the same percentage of water (moisture); otherwise, we should make some proportions. We also recommend paying attention to the calorie density (kcal), as it affects the percentages of the various nutrients and the daily quantities to be administered.

The comparison, therefore, should always be done on the dry substance, which has more or less the same calorie density, or comparisons can be made after calculating the daily quantity to be administered.

High percentages of protein do not necessarily indicate the best product: we must always cross the information and verify the origin of the proteins by reading the ingredients.

Animal proteins, as already mentioned, are qualitatively better than plant proteins and they are more digestible. Corn gluten has a high percentage of protein but a low biological value for our animals; its presence could increase the protein percentage but, being vegetable proteins, from a qualitative point of view it would not be the best.

A high fiber content makes the food less digestible, but we must evaluate the type of fiber present. We have seen that the prebiotic fiber which is present in some ingredients such as beet pulp, chicory, pea fiber etc. can be very useful for gastrointestinal well-being.

Ashes are the minerals present in the food and can derive from supplements or from poor quality ingredients that contain a high amount of bone, such as meat flours or carcasses. In these cases, a low protein content with a high percentage of ash should make us suspicious.

Additives

The term additives refers to added substances other than raw materials. Many are viewed with suspicion, since they are associated with dyes and preservatives, but it is important to know that, with the new European legislation, vitamins, minerals, some amino acids such as taurine, defined as "nutritional additives" also fall into the additives category. Other additives such as chicory extract are called "organoleptic additives". Only the additives presented in a register (the Register of Feed Additives) can be added in foods and there is an obligation to declare them if there is a maximum limit.

Foods, plants and other toxic substances

There are so many dangers at home for our four-legged friends! Plants, drugs, some foods and other chemicals are often the protagonists of various poisonings /intoxications. The severity of the poisoning depends on several factors:
- quantity ingested (dose);
- weight and age of the animal;
- type of substance;
- time and method of contact.

Toxic plants

Potentially toxic plants are various. Among these, there are plants with very common names, while others seem less known but in reality they are very common in homes: the oleander (*Nerium oleander*), the spurge like the castor (*Ricinus communis*), the araceae like the caladium and the calla, calicanto (*Calycanthus*) or winter flower, horse chestnut (*Aesculus hippocastanum*), azalea and rhododendron (*Rhododendron*), cycas (*Cycas revoluta*), poinsettia (*Euphorbia pulcherrima*), kalanchoe, cotyledon, narcissus etc.

Toxicity is often linked to the whole plant, as in the case of the oleander, or only to parts of it: flowers, roots, fruits, leaves and sap, as in the case of the poinsettia. Sialorrhea (hypersalivation), vomiting and diarrhea are the first signs that appear after ingestion. Other symptoms that may appear are: erythema, edema, tremors, convulsions, hepatic necrosis, jaundice, hemolytic anemia and, in severe cases, coma and death.

Toxic drugs

Antipyretics such as paracetamol or the very common *Aspirin* are often used by the owners, as they are considered harmless. Sometimes they are left unattended and are ingested by the animal. They are very toxic and, unfortunately, also very inviting for our pets. They can cause severe abdominal pain, hyperthermia, hyperpnea, anemia, jaundice, cyanosis, coma and death.

Toxic foods

Avocado, garlic, onion, grapes and even chocolate can be harmful. Onion contains a very toxic substance for our pets which is called n-propyl disulfide. It initially causes vomiting and diarrhea; after 1-4 days, hyperthermia, depression, dark coloring of the urine and hemolytic anemia that can be fatal also appear.

Chocolate contains some substances called methylxanthines. One of these is theobromine which, if consumed in large quantities, can be toxic (toxicity, however, is more frequent in dogs than in cats). Within 4-5 hours of intake, vomiting, diarrhea, labored breathing, urinary incontinence and muscle tremors may appear, which, in very severe cases, develop into convulsions and death.

Factors such as individual sensitivity to theobromine, the presence of other foods in the gastrointestinal tract at the time of ingestion and a different amount of theobromine in different chocolate products can cause wide variations in poisoning.

Other toxic substances

These are insecticides, rodenticides, herbicides, antifreeze for engines (ethylene glycol). The latter causes one of the most frequent intoxications in our animals, both for the easy contact our pets can have with the substance (which are not properly disposed or are left unattended) and for its sweet taste and the small amount necessary to prove fatal (1.44 mL/kg). Initially it causes vomiting, diarrhea, lethargy and tremors; later signs are those of a very serious renal failure.

Prevention is certainly the most important thing, so educating the owner is essential. In case of poisoning, the rapidity of the intervention is fundamental, as is collecting a detailed history. Sometimes, unfortunately, this is not possible and in case of doubt it is appropriate to induce vomiting, administer adsorbents and keep the animal under close observation.

Chapter 4

Food management during pathologies

First of all, eat!

OBJECTIVES OF THIS CHAPTER
• Choosing the best diet for each animal and for each pathology   • Choosing the best palatable diet to administer to the pet

In this chapter we will deal with food management during the most frequent pathologies. Many of them, although not all of them, can be influenced by diet, both directly (the pathologies where nutrition can prevent or slow the progression, contain or alleviate the symptoms, etc.) and indirectly (the pathologies associated with hyporexia or anorexia, involving side effects related to an inadequate calorie intake).

In particular, we will discuss the chronic renal failure, gastroenteropathies, the prevention and management of lower urinary tract diseases, obesity, food intolerance/allergy and the heart diseases. We will see what the characteristics of a dedicated plan must be for each animal and for each pathology, in the stage in which it is found.

Obviously, this discussion cannot be exhaustive or replace the experience and knowledge of the specialist. If in doubt, we recommend going to a dedicated center or a to a qualified nutritionist. Sometimes we are so attentive to the diagnosis and administration of the correct drugs and diets that we lose sight of the animal and the owner.

It is evident that focusing the attention on the latter is always important, but in this case, the compliance can make the difference. Sometimes it is necessary to make a compromise in order to always have the situation under control and avoid "do-it-yourself" as much as possible. This way we can limit the damage which, in this case, can be irreversible and fatal.

Chronic renal failure (CRF)

Dietary therapy during CRF represents the cornerstone of the treatment of this pathology. With the diet, we can slow down the progression of kidney damage, reduce the clinical symptoms related above all to uremia, control electrolytes and metabolic disorders and, in particular, we can control the nutritional needs.

Water is essential in order to avoid dehydration and therefore, despite the compensatory polydipsia implemented by the organism, we recommend using wet foods (70-80%) or adding water/broth to the food. The use of multiple bowls or drinking fountains can be another valid solution, especially for cats.

Animals must receive the right amount of energy to prevent the catabolism of the endogenous proteins, which leads to malnutrition and worsening of uremia (Table 4.1). The energy must come from carbohydrates and especially from fats which, in addition to making the food more palatable, increase the energy density, which allows the intake of a reduced volume of food, reducing the symptoms of nausea and vomiting.

The restriction of proteins is recommended in the early stages, especially to slow down the progression of the disease; in the more advanced stages, to control uremic symptoms (Tables 4.2 and 4.3). The IRIS (International Renal Interest Society) recommends a higher restriction of proteins in the presence of proteinuria, especially in stage I of CRF in dogs and cats with UP/UC (urinary protein/creatinine ratio) greater than 2 and also in stages II-IV , starting from a UP/UC higher than 0.5 in dogs and 0.4 in cats.

■ **TABLE 4.1 - THE MULTIPLICATION CONSTANT FOR THE LOAD OF NEEDM IN DOGS AND CATS WITH CRF**

MER multiplication constant in dogs	MER multiplication constant in cats
$MER = 110 \times (\text{weight in kg})^{0.75} \times K$	$MER = 70 \times (\text{weight in kg})^{0.75} \times K$
$K = 1.1\text{-}1.6$	$K = 1.1\text{-}1.4$

■ **TABLE 4.2 - RECOMMENDED PROTEIN PERCENTAGES IN DOGS WITH CRF AND PROTEINURIA**

Recommended protein % in the dog's diet in the DM	Recommended protein % in the dog's diet with proteinuria in the DM
14-20	14-15

DM = dry matter.

■ **TABLE 4.3 - RECOMMENDED PROTEIN PERCENTAGES IN CATS WITH CRF AND PROTEINURIA**

Recommended protein % in the cat's diet in the DM	Recommended protein % in the cat's diet with proteinuria in the DM
28-35	28-30

DM = dry matter.

If the protein restriction is effective, there will be a reduction in urea nitrogen (BUN, Blood Urea Nitrogen) up to 50% within 3-4 weeks. For this reason, it is important to re-evaluate the animal to check whether a further decrease is necessary.

Protein restriction can lead to malnutrition, with loss of muscle mass, decreased immune response and a decreased synthesis of hemoglobin and proteins. For this reason, it is important to monitor the animal and implement a gradual restriction, possibly comparing the available diets. The major restriction is recommended in stages III and IV and the proteins must be of high quality to avoid deficiencies in essential amino acids.

The reduction of phosphorus is essential to control hyperphosphataemia and secondary renal hyperparathyroidism, with all the alterations related to it: hypocalcaemia, osteodystrophy, reduction of vitamin D_3 (Table 4.4).

■ **TABLE 4.4 - RECOMMENDED PHOSPHORUS LEVELS IN DIFFERENT STAGES**

Stage	Recommended phosphorus blood levels in dogs and cats (IRIS)
II	2.7-4.6 mg/dL
III	<5 mg/dL
IV	<6 mg/dL

IRIS = International Renal Interest Society.

The first thing to do is to reduce the diet intake of phosphorus, decreasing the protein intake and using proteins with a lower phosphorus concentration (for example chicken breast, chicken eggs). If this is not enough, intestinal chelators (calcium acetate, calcium carbonate or lanthanum) are used, which must be mixed with the meal (Table 4.5). The use of chelators can have some contraindications (hypophosphataemia, hypercalcaemia, gastrointestinal problems), therefore their use is recommended to start gradually, prescribing dedicated diets that do not contain them, introducing them on later stages. Phosphatemia should be initially monitored every 4-5 weeks, then every 3-4 months.

Hypokalaemia can appear mainly in cats, although not at all of them. It is generally of a moderate degree, with no obvious symptoms. In dogs, sometimes, hyperkalaemia may occur especially in animals which are fed with commercial renal diets, since they are generally more integrated with this element. For this reason, it is important to always check the concentration of potassium present in the diet and, if necessary, use home prepared diets, prepared by a qualified nutritionist, if you are unable to control the blood level of the potassium.

The restriction of sodium has always been recommended, since the remaining nephrons are not sufficiently able to expel it. Sodium accumulates and contributes to hypertension, but it is important to know that its reduction is not able to lower the blood pressure (Table 4.6). Hypertension is frequent in the CRF and it is one of the factors responsible for the progression of the disease, therefore it is important to monitor it and intervene if necessary. Keeping the blood pressure within the recommended limits also allows us to better control the proteinuria and therefore to use a higher percentage of protein in the diet.

■ TABLE 4.5 - **RECOMMENDED PHOSPHORUS LEVELS IN THE FOOD OF DOGS AND CATS IN THE DM**

Recommended phosphorus levels in the dog's diet in % in the DM	Recommended phosphorus levels in the cat's diet in % in the DM
0.2-0.5	0.3-0.6

DM = dry matter.

■ TABLE 4.6 - **RECOMMENDED SODIUM LEVELS IN THE FOOD OF DOGS AND CATS IN THE DM**

Recommended sodium levels in the dog's diet in % in the DM	Recommended sodium levels in the cat's diet in % in the DM
<0.3	<0.4

DM = dry matter.

One of the alterations which is present especially in stages III and IV is the metabolic acidosis, linked both to the reduction of the elimination of hydrogen ions by the kidney and to the reduction of the reabsorption of the bicarbonates. Metabolic acidosis increases the catabolism, the degradation of muscle proteins and the bone demineralization, therefore it is important to control it with the use of alkalisers (for example calcium bicarbonate, sodium citrate).

However, the use of these substances can aggravate some clinical symptoms such as lethargy, anorexia, vomiting and nausea, therefore it is clear that it is necessary to check their need before prescribing them, choosing the diet also based on this factor. Long-chain omega-3 fatty acids, such as eicosapentaenoic acid (EPA) and docosahexaenoic acid (DHA), have a protective action for the kidney and they reduce the glomerular pressure and proteinuria, slowing down the progression of the disease (Table 4.7).

Fermentable fibers are also very useful: as we know, they promote intestinal bacterial multiplication. Bacteria use ammonia nitrogen to grow, even that comes from food proteins; in this way they reduce the availability and therefore the absorption.

In humans and rats, it has been demonstrated a reduction of the urea in the blood thanks to the ingestion of these fibers. It can be assumed, even though the studies are lacking, that the same mechanism also occurs in dogs and cats.

Oxidative damage is considered one of the causes and it is among those causes which are responsible for the progression of various pathologies: cancer, atherosclerosis, cardiovascular diseases, diabetes mellitus. Free radicals are also considered risk factors for the progression of the CRF. The use of antioxidants such as vitamin E, vitamin C, lutein etc. is very useful for reducing kidney damage (tubulointerstitial changes, proteinuria, glomerulosclerosis) (Table 4.8). However, the quantities and synergy between the different antioxidants have yet to be clarified and defined.

The diet plays a fundamental role for the CRF, but it must be used appropriately. CRF is a progressive and dynamic disease, therefore the diet must be

■ **TABLE 4.7 - RECOMMENDED OMEGA-3 LEVELS FOR FOOD AND THE RELATIONSHIP BETWEEN OMEGA-3 AND OMEGA-6**

Recommended EPA-DHA % in the dog's diet in the DM	Recommended EPA-DHA % in the cat's diet in the DM
0.4-2.5	0.4-2.5
Omega-6/Omega-3 ratio = 1:1/7:1	

DM = dry matter.

▦ TABLE 4.8 - QRECOMMENDED QUANTITIES OF VITAMINS E, C IN DOGS AND IN CATS WITH CRF

Vitamins	Dogs	Cats
E	400 IU/kg	500 IU/kg
C	100 IU/kg	100-200 IU/kg

modified and adapted over time according to the stage of the disease and the metabolic state of the patient. It is recommended starting from stage II, also to get the animal used to the new diet when there are still no symptoms such as nausea or vomiting.

In the II and III stages, the primary objective is slowing down the progression of the disease; in stage IV the main objective is to alleviate the symptoms linked to uremia. Checks must be frequent, every 2-3 weeks in the first period and, subsequently, at least four times a year.

☞ Which kidney diet should be used?

The renal diets on the market are numerous, but it is necessary to evaluate them from time to time, based on the needs of the animal. You can also consider the possibility of proposing a dedicated home diet, formulated by a qualified nutritionist, especially if the animal does not eat or if it needs a particular diet that is not commercially available.

Multi-prescription in the progress of CRF is not practicable: the diet must be modulated on the animal and over time. As we have seen, it is not necessary to immediately practice excessive protein restriction or use acidifying or chelating substances.

Gastrointestinal pathologies

No other apparatus like the gastrointestinal one, is so directly and immediately influenced by nutrition. The modification of the ingredients, the nutritional profile, the consistency of the food, the method, the time and the frequency of administration represent a valid and powerful tool for the management of these pathologies. Drug therapy without the association of a diet therapy often produces null or only partial results. In some other cases the diet can also be a valid diagnostic tool.

In this chapter we will discuss the most frequent diseases in the veterinary practice and those that make the professionals or owners turn more frequently to a nutritionist, such as acute enteropathies, chronic enteropathies - including diet-responsive enteropathies (Food Responsive Enteropathies, FRE) and those responsive to steroid administration (Steroid Responsive Enteropathies, SRE, or Inflammatory Bowel Diseases, IBD) - and finally colitis.

Acute gastroenteritis

Acute gastroenteritis is among the most common diseases in the veterinary practice. The causes can be different: bacterial, viral, parasitic infections, adverse reactions to food. The diet must supply all the nutrients and it should allow the normalization of intestinal function and motility. Generally, fasting is provided for at least 24-36 hours before starting eating food again, but we know how important it is to start it as soon as possible to preserve the integrity of the mucous membrane and intestinal villi and avoid bacterial translocation. The diet must be highly digestible, with a moderate fat content and a low fiber content (fermentable and non-fermentable) (Table 4.9).

The use of the new antigenic sources is not necessary, but it is recommended, especially when there is a doubt about an adverse reaction to food. Initially the quantity to be administered must be 25% of the RER (Resting Energy Requirements) and then gradually increased ("minimum nutrition"), since the digestion and absorption capacity is compromised.

$$RER = 70 \times (\text{weight in kg})^{0.75} \text{ (dogs and cats)}$$

High-quality home and commercial dry diets are recommended, while regarding wet ones is only partial. In fact, commercial wet diets are often less digestible, with a higher content of both fats, which delay gastric emptying and increase intestinal peristalsis, and of viscous fibers, which alter digestibility and gastrointestinal motility.

■ **TABLE 4.9 - RECOMMENDED LEVELS OF LIPIDM, FIBER AND DIGESIBILITY IN THE FOOD IN THE DM**

Species	% of lipids in the DM	% of fiber in the DM	% digestibility in the DM
Dogs	12-15	<5 mixed	87 proteins >90 fats and carbohydrates
Cats	15-25	<5 mixed	87 proteins >90 fats and carbohydrates

DM = dry matter.

We must always compare and verify diets, as we saw in the previous chapter, especially those dedicated to the gastrointestinal tract.

 Before changing the diet we must always make sure that what our patient is taking is not adequate, in order not to worsen the situation.

Chronic gastritis

Chronic gastritis is one of the most common causes of vomiting in dogs and cats. The causes can be different: parasitic, metabolic disorders (uremia, liver disease), immune-mediated, adverse reactions to food.

Water is an important nutrient, but in the presence of dehydration, fluid therapy obviously becomes necessary, as well as for alterations of chlorine, sodium and potassium, although in the diet it is still appropriate that they are present in greater quantities (Table 4.10).

The proteins must be of high quality, highly digestible, in limited quantities to avoid excessive production of gastrin and acid secretions, preferably antigenically new or hydrolyzed (Table 4.11).

To promote gastric emptying, the fat level must be low (Table 4.12).

The fiber level must be low and soluble fibers such as *psyllium*, gum Arabic, Guar gum, pectin etc. must be avoided, since they make the meal viscous and slow gastric emptying (Table 4.13).

▨ **TABLE 4.10 - RECOMMENDED POTASSIUM, CHLORINE AND SODIUM LEVELS IN THE FOOD IN THE DM**

Species	% of potassium in the DM	% of chlorine in the DM	% of sodium in the DM
Dogs and cats	0.8-1.1	0.5-1.3	0.3-0.5

DM = dry matter.

▨ **TABLE 4.11 - RECOMMENDED PROTEIN LEVELS IN THE FOOD IN THE DM**

Species	% of protein in the DM
Dogs	16-26
Cats	30-40

DM = dry matter.

TABLE 4.12 - RECOMMENDED FAT LEVELS IN THE FOOD IN THE DM

Species	% of lipids in the DM
Dogs	<15
Cats	<25

DM = dry matter.

TABLE 4.13 - RECOMMENDED FIBER LEVELS IN THE FOOD IN THE DM

Species	% of fiber in the DM
Dogs and cats	<5

DM = dry matter.

The home diet or a commercial wet diet are recommended, preferably liquid or semi-liquid but with a low level of fat and fiber. Liquids leave the stomach faster than dry food. The diet must be provided at room temperature or, better, at body temperature (around 38° C).

Inflammatory bowel diseases (IBDs)

Chronic gastroenteritis is a disease characterized by diarrhea, vomiting, nausea and, in severe cases, weight loss. It can be divided into responsive to diet (FRE), antibiotics (ARE) and/or steroids (SRD). Among the most frequent are IBDs, a group of idiopathic diseases characterized by infiltration of lymphocytes, plasma cells, eosinophils, macrophages, neutrophils or combinations of these into the lamina propria. The etiology is not yet fully clarified, but there is a strong suspicion that there is an abnormal immune response from the mucosa to the intestinal bacterial microflora, its products or to the products of the diet.

The diet plays a fundamental role, alone or in association with the drug therapy, reducing irritation and inflammation, changing the bacterial flora and normalizing intestinal motility. Three types of diets can be used: 1) high digestibility diet with low fiber content; 2) high digestibility diet with high fiber content; 3) elimination diet with new antigenic or hydrolyzed sources.

Which approach is better?

The approach depends on several factors and the diet must be tested on the animal. Symptomatology (diarrhea) returns quickly (about 7-10 days); in our experience, a combination of the first and third diet is often the best and the most decisive solution.

Homemade or commercial hydrolyzed elimination diets are recommended, while single-protein commercial diets are less indicated, as several studies have shown different and/or undeclared protein sources on the labels, which could affect the results.

The diet should have a high energy density, to reduce the volume of the meal and, consequently, the distension and gastrointestinal secretions. Unfortunately, the high energy density involves a high presence of fats, which can exacerbate osmotic diarrhea and the loss of proteins. A diet with a moderate energy intake (4-4.5 kcal/g) and with a medium-low level of fats is therefore more appropriate (Table 4.14).

In severe cases or in the presence of lymphangiectasia, a greater lipid restriction should be expected. Also in these cases omega-3 fatty acids can be useful for controlling inflammation:

$$EPA + DHA = 125 \text{ mg/kg/day}$$
$$\text{Omega-6/Omega-3 ratio} = 1:1/3:1$$

The proteins must be of high quality and extremely digestible (>87%), "new" or hydrolyzed and in adequate quantities. Sometimes it is also recommended to use the "sacrificial protein" (which is a new protein) in the first phase (6 weeks) and to replace it with another protein, always a new one, when the inflammation of the intestine is under control and the mucosa is healing, so as to avoid further sensitization. If the animal is under cortisone treatment, it is preferable to make the change before stopping the drug or reducing the dosage (Table 4.15).

▦ TABLE 4.14 - RECOMMENDED FAT LEVELS IN THE FOOD IN THE DM

Species	% of lipids in the DM
Dogs	12-15
Cats	15-25

DM = dry matter.

▦ TABLE 4.15 - RECOMMENDED PROTEIN LEVELS IN THE FOOD IN THE DM

Species	% of protein in the DM
Dogs	25
Cats	35

DM = dry matter.

It is recommended to use a low amount of fiber, to avoid reducing the energy density and digestibility of the food (see Table 4.13).

A deficiency of vitamin B_{12}, folate, vitamin K and zinc can frequently be present. If the animal responds to therapy, integration with the diet may be sufficient, but in severe cases or in the absence of response to therapy, parenteral intervention is necessary.

Colitis
Alessia Candellone

The large intestine, and in particular the colon, can be affected by numerous diseases that require different nutritional approaches. Considering the predominant role played by the diet in the management of *chronic enteropathies* of the large intestine, the causes of which are summarized in Table 4.16, attention will be focused on these disorders.

A common aspect of the various colopathies, however, is the clinical manifestation of the "colic" patient, whose main sign is the diarrhea of the large intestine, that is characterized by mucoid feces, produced with increased frequency but in reduced volume, occasionally characterized by blood streaks of bright red color, superficial, mainly affecting the last part of faecal production. The subject may also display tenesmus, dyschezia, vomiting and, in severe or ongoing cases of colon cancer, weight loss and reduction of BCS. It is not uncommon for patients with functional or colonic motility disorders to also have constipation.

In this section, our attention will be focused on the chronic colitis that recognizes a dietary (adverse food reaction colitis, FRE, and fibro-responsive colitis) or immune (large intestine IBD) cause as the trigger. The considerations set out regarding the etiopathogenesis and the criteria for choosing the protein sources in progress for FRE for the small intestine also apply to the large intestine.

■ **TABLE 4.16 - CLASSIFICATION OF CHRONIC ENTEROPATHIES OF THE LARGE INTESTINE**

Conditions that cause chronic large intestine enteropathy
Adverse reactions to food (FRE of the large intestine)
Fiber-responsive colitis
Irritable bowel syndrome (IBS)
IBD of the large intestine (lymphoplasmacytic colitis, eosinophilic colitis, granulomatous colitis, histiocytic-ulcerative colitis)
Colon cancer (adenomas, adenocarcinomas, lymphomas, leiomyomas etc.)
Functional pathologies, from dysmotility

Here we will instead provide more details on the choice of fibrous ingredients (see below, *Irritable bowel syndrome, [IBS]*).

During chronic colitis, regardless of the underlying cause, three types of dietary approaches can be adopted and implemented in an order which is deemed the most appropriate based on the presentation of the individual patient:

1. Diets enriched in fiber.
2. Diets containing highly digestible and low residue foods.
3. Elimination dietary trials.

In subjects characterized by mild and intermittent symptoms (see below, *Irritable bowel syndrome, [IBS]*), dietary fiber supplementation can be suggested without changing the patient's original diet. The optimal level of fiber inclusion in the diet and the type of approach to be used can only be determined by trial and error.

In fact, there are no clinical alterations or ancillary tests capable of predicting which method will be successful, but numerous dietary trials are often necessary to understand which diet works best in a specific case. If you opt for an elimination diet plan, a new and exclusive source of animal protein, with high digestibility, or a protein hydrolyzate must be associated with a single source of starches and the introduction of adequate portions of soluble and insoluble fiber.

All other possible dietary sources of protein and carbohydrates should be eliminated, including chews, snacks and premiums, vitamin-mineral supplements, dietary supplements and/or flavored medications.

The key nutritional factors to take in consideration in the selection of dry or wet commercial foods or in the formulation of homemade diets for patients with chronic large intestine enteropathy are summarized in Table 4.17.

Irritable bowel syndrome (IBS)

Irritable bowel syndrome (IBS) is a disorder that is currently still poorly defined in dogs, which causes the appearance of diarrhea of the large intestine, for which no significant histological lesions or causative etiological agents have been identified. It represents the canine equivalent of human irritable bowel syndrome, once also defined with the names of *spastic colon, nervous colon* and *spastic colitis*.

It is a very common and highly debilitating condition in humans, affecting about 10% of the global population, with a higher incidence in women and between the ages of 20 and 50. Despite the high prevalence, the etiopatho-

◼ TABLE 4.17 - MAIN NUTRITIONAL FACTORS FOR MANAGEMENT OF CHOLITIS*

Nutrients	Recommended levels
Proteins**	Adult dogs: 18-30% Growing dogs: 25-32% Adult cats: 30-45% Growing cats: 35-50%
Fats	Adult dogs: 815% Adult cats: 9-25%
Total fiber	High digestibility diets: <5% Fiber enriched diets: 7-8%
Electrolytes	Sodium: 0.3-0.5% Chlorine: 0.5-1.3% Potassium: 0.8-1.1%

DM = dry matter.
*The values are expressed as % on the DM.
**NB: consider using elimination diets or protein hydrolysates.

genesis is currently still partially unknown and probably multifactorial. The similarities between dogs and humans, first of all the possible influence of the environment on the clinical manifestations of the pathology, have identified the canine patient as a possible spontaneous model for the study of this pathology in other species.

IBS in dogs, in fact, represents a frequent cause of chronic recurrent diarrhea of the large intestine in young, hyperactive or stressed animals. The affected subjects do not show other extraintestinal anomalies and the colon is normal in endoscopic and histological examinations; therefore, irritable bowel syndrome has been counted among functional disorders. The condition is presumed to recognize a neurological component, with motor or sensory alteration of the colon, although the scientific evidence supporting this hypothesis in dogs is currently scarce.

The symptomatological corollary varies from subject to subject, both in terms of the frequency and severity of the symptoms manifested. Intermittent episodes of mucoid stools, hematochezia, flatulence, tenesmus and nausea are described. As previously mentioned, it is a pathology of difficult diagnostic confirmation, therefore before issuing a diagnosis of IBS it would be advisable to research and exclude all the other causes of diarrhea of the large intestine (parasitic, toxic, dietetic causes, etc.).

Since dietary fibers are able to modulate parameters such as myoelectric activity, motility, faecal volume, gastrointestinal transit time and microbiota, dietary fiber supplementation is often recommended in human and canine patients. Scientific studies have shown that a large number of subjects suffering from IBS can benefit from the inclusion of 1-5% of insoluble fibers (dry matter) and 10-15% of soluble fiber in the DM. Foods integrated with mixed fiber sources (soluble and insoluble) at levels between 5 and 10% in the DM would also seem to be adequate for the food management of the disease.

In daily practice, however, it is not always possible to know the content of the different fiber fractions contained in commercial food or in vegetable raw material; therefore, it is customary to formulate or prescribe diets in which the *raw fiber* content of the diet, expressed in the DM, is within 8%. In this case, the list of fibrous foods shown on the label will guide the choice, thus suggesting the relative soluble or insoluble fiber content.

Food sources of insoluble fiber are, for example, cellulose, hemicellulose and lignins, while high portions of soluble fiber can be found in pectins, gums and *psyllium* seeds. Whole grains such as rice, oats and wheat, pea fiber and beet pulp represent mixed fiber sources, widely used for the formulation of homemade or commercial diets for the management of fibro-responsive colitis and IBS.

A practical approach is therefore to prescribe or formulate a diet containing mixed fiber sources (soluble and insoluble), selecting ingredients such as wheat or oat bran to subsequently consider food sources of soluble fiber (for example *psyllium* powder) in case of failure of the therapeutic response. Foods other than those selected for the control of clinical symptoms should be strictly prohibited, especially in subjects in which the sudden and frequent dietary changes, the intake of snacks and treats or access to leftovers from the kitchen may constitute or trigger the appearance of colitic episodes.

If concomitant pathologies do not allow the dog's diet to be modified in terms of the type of food and/or the relationship between nutrients, it is possible to administer dietary supplements of soluble or mixed fibers. Soluble fibers, for example, can be added to the diet in the form of *psyllium* powder, with a starting dose of 1.3 g of *psyllium* powder/kg of body weight, corresponding to about 6 teaspoons for a 15 kg dog.

Soluble fibers, in fact, are able to improve the quality and consistency of the stool, supporting the production of butyrate for the health of the colonocytes.

However, it is not able to intervene sufficiently on the possible intestinal dysmotility, and in this case, the use of complementary foods integrated with insoluble fibers or food sources of insoluble fibers may be necessary. Many homemade diets formulated for dogs with IBS provide for the inclusion of whole grains, usually dedicated to human breakfast, in doses equal to 1 teaspoon for every 13-15 kg of body weight. Insoluble fibers, in fact, have the ability to bind water, increase fecal mass and improve intestinal motility. The administration of more than 5 teaspoons in subjects with a body weight <15 kg is not recommended.

Regardless of the selected dietary sources of fiber, the addition of fibers should be done systematically and it should be modulated based on the patient's clinical response. The integration should take place gradually, with increments of about 25% compared to the initial dose, every 2 weeks, until we achieve the minimum dose sufficient to improve or resolve the gastrointestinal symptoms. In some rare cases, the addition of dietary fiber may exacerbate the frequency and severity of clinical signs; in this case the dietary supplement should be immediately suspended, as it is unlikely that in the event of an initial worsening, improvements will be obtained over time.

Alongside nutritional management, various pharmacological protocols have been proposed for the management of IBS, which however fall outside the scope of this volume.

Finally, given the frustration that owners often feel about the condition of their pet, it is essential to establish a good communicative relationship with them in order to guarantee their collaboration during the entire diagnostic and therapeutic process.

Lower urinary tract diseases

These diseases are frequently found in our animals. In dogs, the incidence increases with the increasing of age and the conditions are mostly related to *bacterial infections* and *urolithiasis. Idiopathic cystitis* and urolithiasis are frequent in cats which are less than 10 years old; in older cats, as well as in dogs, bacterial infections are the most frequent.

Urolithiasis
Urolithiasis accounts for up to about 45% of the causes of these diseases. Several factors are involved: familiar, congenital and/or acquired factors. Among the most important factors are the supersaturation of the urine, the retention or

reduction of urinary transit, the lack of inhibitors or the presence of promoters for the formation and growth of uroliths. About 90% of urolithiasis is represented by struvite and calcium oxalate; purines are less frequent, with about 5-8% of cases (urates, urate salts such as ammonium urate and xanthines etc.) and cystine, with about 1% (Tables 4.18 and 4.19).

Struvite

Struvite crystals and uroliths are composed of phosphate, ammonium and magnesium and they can be formed in the presence or absence of urinary tract infections. The presence of sterile struvite is typical of cats under 10 years old and generally affects both males and females in the same percentage. Struvite is formed both because of the composition of the cat's diet which is naturally rich in phosphate, ammonium and magnesium, and because the cat produces concentrated (supersaturated) urine, and also the pH of the urine can rise naturally after meals following the "tide" postprandial alkaline "(Box 4.1), causing the precipitation of these minerals.

▦ **TABLE 4.18 - SUMMARY OF THE MOST IMPORTANT FACTORS TO TAKE INTO CONSIDERATION IN ORDER TO PREVENT UROLITHASIS**

Important common factors	Feline idiopathic cystitis	Struvite	Calcium oxalate	Purines	Cysteine
Water	Wet food	Wet food	Wet food	Wet food	Wet food
Specific weight	–	<1,025 in dogs <1,035 in cats	<1,025 in dogs <1,035 in cat	<1,025 in dogs <1,035 in cats	<1,025 in dogs <1,035 in cats
pH	–	<6.6	>7	>7	>7.5
Proteins	–	To increase	To decrease	To decrease	To decrease

▦ **TABLE 4.19 - COMPARISON BETWEEN DRY FOOD AND WET FOOD ON WATER INTAKE AND ON URINARY PRODUCTION IN CATS**

Volume (mL/day)	Wet food	Dry food
Food's water	246	6
Drinking water	32	221
Total water intake	278	227
Fecal water	27	44
Urine	166	79

From: Burger IH, Smith PM. Effects of diet on the urine characteristics of the cat. In: Edney ATB (Ed.) *Nutrition, Malnutrition and Dietetics in the Dog and Cat: Proceedings of an international symposium;* 1987 Sept 3-4; Hanover, Germany. British Veterinary Association UK, pp. 71-73.

BOX 4.1 THE POSTPRANDIAL ALKALINE TIDE

The postprandial alkaline tide is caused by renal compensation which, in order to keep a constant pH of body fluids following the loss of hydrogen during the meal, eliminates alkaline ions (bicarbonates) in the urine causing an increase in pH. It is directly proportional to the amount of the meal and the presence of alkalizing or acidifying substances or ingredients in the diet.

Precisely for the presence of the postprandial alkaline tide, for a correct assessment of the urinary pH, it is essential that the animal has been fasting for at least 8-12 hours.

To prevent the formation of struvite stones, it is fundamental to first carry out the "dilution" of the urine [specific gravity (SG) lower than 1,035-1,040 in cats and 1,025 in dogs], the pH should be below 6.6 and the diet should contain high quality animal proteins (naturally acidifying because they are rich in sulfur amino acids) with a low carbohydrate content (naturally alkalizing because they are rich in potassium salts). The diet should have a moderate magnesium content (0.04-0.14%), less than/equal to 0.25%. It is also possible to obtain the dissolution of this type of crystals and stones in 2-4 weeks with the restriction of phosphorus, magnesium and proteins, bringing the pH around the value of 6.

Dedicated wet commercial diets or homemade diets formulated by a nutritionist are recommended; the dry commercial ones are less indicated, even if they are dietetic, as they are "dry" (8-10% of water). In any case, the addition of acidifying substances in commercial diets formulated for these problems should be avoided, to avoid the side effects related to hyperacidosis; dry diets enriched with salt (sodium chloride) should also be used with caution to increase the water intake and therefore the volume of urine, for any side effects that sodium can cause (increased risk of formation of calcium oxalate stones and worsening of blood urea nitrogen). For the same reason, the use of loop diuretics is not recommended.

Struvite urolithiasis can also be induced by infections due to the presence of urease-producing bacteria; these are more typical in dogs and mostly in females, while in cats they are more present in individuals less than one year old.

The composition of the diet is not important for prevention, but even in this case dissolution can be induced, which usually occurs slower (about 70 days). It is essential to continue with antibiotic treatment throughout the dissolution period, because the bacteria can be trapped in the matrix and are gradually released into the urine by perpetuating the cycle.

Calcium oxalates

These crystals or stones are composed precisely of oxalates and calcium. They are frequent especially in dogs, mainly in males. They cannot be dissolved, therefore prevention is even more important, especially in predisposed subjects such as the obese individuals. There are several things to do: 1) dilution of urine to reduce saturation and increase urinary transit (SG <1,025 in dogs; SG 1,035 in cats); 2) reduce the presence of the two elements with the use of inhibitors such as citrate and magnesium, or their precursors (for example oxalic acid, end product of the metabolism of vitamin C, serine, glycine which forms an insoluble salt with calcium), or avoiding hypercalciuria, hypercalcaemia, metabolic acidosis (cause of hypercalciuria), excess and/or activation of vitamin D (for example due to a lack of phosphorus) for the hypercalcaemia that follows; 3) maintain the pH >7 to avoid the formation of oxalates.

We should pay attention to commercial maintenance diets that advertise benefits for the urinary tract: generally, they are diets that promote urine acidification, have a low magnesium content and can be valid for animals predisposed to struvite stones but not for those predisposed to oxalate calculosis.

Purines

Purines are catabolites (hypoxanthines, xanthines, uric acid, uric acid salts, etc.) which are components of DNA and RNA. They can be of endogenous origin or derive from the diet. Among purine uroliths, ammonium urate urolites are the most frequent. They are formed from uric acid and ammonium and are often secondary to vascular anomalies. They are also frequent in some breeds such as Dalmatians, in dogs, or Shorthair, in cats. In dogs it is possible to attempt dissolution with dilution (SG <1,025) and restriction of proteins and purines, bringing the pH above 7 and administering allopurinol.

In cats, as there are not an adequate number of studies, surgical stone removal is the only option for the moment. Obviously, prevention is essential. Commercial renal diets, for their composition and characteristics, can be recommended, as well as homemade diets, if they are well formulated. The restriction of purines, in the case of administration of allopurinol, is important since allopurinol can predispose to the formation of xanthine uroliths due to the accumulation of xanthines following the lack of degradation. Allopurinol should be used carefully in animals with kidney problems, as it may worsen the kidney function.

Cystine

Cystine crystals or stones are the least frequent in our pets. Both male and female cats are affected, while in dogs, males are the most predisposed. High concentrations of cystine are present when there is an alteration of the absorption in the proximal renal tubule. For dogs, there is a medical protocol for their dissolution using thiopronin-based drugs (2-MPG) at a dose of 15 mg/kg per os every 12 hours, while for cats there are insufficient studies. For prevention, the increase in pH above 7.5 and the dilution of specific gravity below 1,025 are indicated, together with the reduction in the amount of protein.

Idiopathic cystitis

Idiopathic cystitis is among the most common causes of diseases of the lower urinary tract, which generally affect cats under 10 years old. They are characterized by hematuria, pollakiuria, stranguria and inappropriate urination. The causes have not yet been clarified, but there seems to be a strong stress-related component. For this reason, together with the use of wet diets (there are no other special indications for the diet), environmental enrichment and in any case general attention to the environment in which the cat lives are recommended (for example an adequate number of bowls, a higher number of litters than the number of cats etc.).

Bacterial infections

They are common, especially in older animals, in both dogs and cats. Dietary factors that can be put in place to prevent these infections have not yet been highlighted. The involved bacteria manage to survive in a pH ranging from 4 to 9, therefore it is useless to make changes in this sense. Some studies demonstrate the usefulness of probiotics, in particular MOS, which in vitro limits the adhesion of *Escherichia coli* to the epithelium of the urinary tract. Probably, also in this case, the dilution of the urine and the increase of the urinary transit can be useful for their management.

Overweight and obesity

Natalia Russo

Obesity is one of the main nutritional disorders in dogs and cats. Although some diseases, such as hypothyroidism and hyperadrenocorticism, or drugs, such as glucocorticoids and anticonvulsants, may be the cause, the main reason for the development of obesity is the positive difference between energy intake and energy expenditure. Therefore, excessive dietary intake or inadequate use of energy can lead to a positive energy balance state and therefore to weight gain.

Obesity is defined as an accumulation of excessive amounts of adipose tissue in the body which is over 20% of the ideal weight.

Several studies report that the incidence of overweight/obesity in the canine population is 22-40%, even reaching 56% in Europe. The incidence of feline obesity is similar to that of dogs and in both species obesity is increasing.

There are several predisposing factors to consider: genetics, sterilization, dietary and behavioral factors (the owner).

Genetic predisposition is one of the primary factors. We have seen how working breeds, selected to live in cold countries, such as Retrievers and Nordic breeds (Alaskan Malamute), or some breeds of cats (Domestic Shorthair), have lower energy needs, about 20% less than a hunting dog of the same weight. This explains why it is not unusual to see an overweight/obese Labrador Retriever on the street.

Sterilization is another important factor, since it would lead to a decrease in the metabolic rate of about 20% due to a reduction in sex hormones, which leads to an increase in food intake and a reduction in physical activity, without a corresponding reduction of energy intake.

Dietary factors can lead to the development of obesity in both species and this seems to be related to the consumption of too fatty meals, but above all to the intake of treats and/or extra meals.

Behavioral factors are among the most important to cause the development of obesity, in which the "owner" element plays a primary role.

For cats, possible factors involved in the development of obesity include anxiety, depression, an inability to establish proper eating behavior and an inability to develop satiety control, commonly referred to as feline bulimia. The owner-animal relationship is important and has proven more intense in obese cat owners.

The owner's incorrect interpretation of feline behavior is important; regarding this, many owners misread their cat's behavioral signs associated with food. Unlike humans and dogs, for whom eating is a social function, cats have no intrinsic need for social interaction during feeding moments. When the cat begins the contact, owners often think it is a food request even when it isn't.

However, if food is supplied at such times, the cat soon learns that initiating contact leads to a food reward; this, in fact, is a common element with childhood obesity (recent studies take obese cats as a model to understand the phenomenon of childhood obesity).

For dogs, however, behavioral factors are mainly related to how the owner sees food. Often the owners observe the dog while he eats and, if he does not finish the food, they think that it is not a welcome food and therefore they tend to change it for something more palatable and unfortunately they often choose a fatter diet. If an owner has an unbalanced diet and a predisposition to obesity, it has been seen that his pet will also be overweight/obese.

As in humans, obesity also increases the risk of mortality in dogs and cats and can predispose to numerous diseases (Table 4.20).

 How is obesity measured?
The simplest method, although not precise because it is still subjective, is to evaluate it through the BCS (see Chapter 2, Figure 2.1).

Obesity treatment
In humans, current therapeutic options for obesity include diet management, exercise, psychological and behavioral modification, drug therapy and surgery. In dogs and cats above the indicated methods are:
- diet therapy, with reduction of kcal and modification of ingredients;
- physical exercise.

 How do you calculate the daily requirement of an obese animal?
The formulas for calculating the maintenance energy can be multiplied by a coefficient of 0.8, to reduce daily calories by 20%:

■ **TABLE 4.20 - DISEASES ASSOCIATED WITH OBESITY IN PETS**

Metabolic abnormalities	• Hyperlipidemia/Dyslipidemia • Insulin resistance • Glucose intolerance • Metabolic syndrome • Liver lipidosis (cats)
Endocrinopathies	• Hyperadrenocorticism • Hypothyroidism • Diabetes mellitus • Insulinoma • Hypopituitarism • Hypothalamic lesions
Orthopedic disorders	• Osteoarthritis • Humeral fractures of the condyle • Cruciate ligament rupture • Hernias of the disc • Joint disorders
Cardiorespiratory diseases	• Tracheal collapse • Airway obstruction • Laryngeal paralysis • Heart failure • Dyspnea • Hypertension
Urogenital system	• Urinary incontinence • Urolithiasis • Infertility • Complications of childbirth
Neoplasms	• Bladder • Breast
Other	• Increased anesthetic risk • Exercise intolerance • Heat intolerance • Decreased lifespan

$$\text{MER in dogs} = 110 \times (\text{weight in kg})^{0.75} \times 0.8$$
$$\text{MER in cats} = 70 \times (\text{weight in kg})^{0.75} \times 0.8$$

Dietary management has changed over the years; in fact, in the past, the intake of insoluble fiber (scarcely digestible) in meals was increased, in order to always maintain the same volume but a lower calorie intake.

This approach was not suitable for all the patients, especially in dog breeds that are more predisposed to obesity and in some cases in cats. Today the mostly used and mostly recommended approach is the stimulation of the metabolism. This can be obtained by increasing the protein intake above 40% of the dry matter, in order to activate a lipomobilization from the adipose tissues. However, the advice, as always, is to adapt the weight reduction protocol to the individual patient and to its general state of health.

Additional dietary factors that may be useful for weight loss include the integration of L-carnitine and conjugated linoleic acid (CLA), but regarding the latter, conflicting data are reported.

L-carnitine is an amino acid which is synthesized in the liver and kidneys by lysine and methionine in the presence of ascorbate. The dietary supplement of L-carnitine improves nitrogen retention, increasing lean body mass and reducing fat mass. The incorporation of L-carnitine at a level of 50-300 ppm in weight loss diets has been shown to limit the loss of lean tissue during weight loss. The possible mechanisms of this protective effect on lean tissues include the improvement of the oxidation of fatty acids and the availability of energy for protein synthesis in times of need.

CLA belongs to a family of isomers of fatty acids derived from linoleic acid. Various experimental animal studies have suggested that it has an antiadipogenic effect; the proposed mechanisms include inhibiting the activity of stearoyl-CoA 9-desaturase, which limits the synthesis of monounsaturated fatty acids through the synthesis of triglycerides and the suppression of the lengthening and desaturation of fatty acids into long-chain fatty acids.

 What is the weight that an animal can and should lose?

As a rule, an animal must lose 0.5-2% of its weight per week. This allows you to control the weight loss and to estimate the necessary time. Once the animal has reached its ideal weight, the kcal and the diet must be reshaped in order to maintain the achieved weight.

 Which diet to choose?

There are several commercial diets, both wet and dry, which are complete and balanced, designed precisely to achieve weight loss and they are integrated so that the animal does not end up with nutrient deficiency. In fact, for an animal it is not possible to have a diet with a maintenance food, since reducing the kcal also reduces all the other nutrients. In general, it is always advisable to calculate the daily needs for each animal based on the chosen product.

If you want to rely on the indicated tables, you must keep in mind that the quantities to be given are those relating to the ideal weight and not to the current one. Well formulated home diets can also be used with excellent results. The latter are to be taken into consideration especially when the animal/ owner relationship is expressed only or mainly through food. It is also essential to predict and calculate treats and snacks in the diet.

Obesity is one of the diseases with the highest therapeutic failure and the highest recurrence rate. An obese person is said to remain so throughout their life, even if they maintain a perfect weight, so it is important that the owners change the animal's eating habits and that they do not feel like they have to spoil their pets because they love them.

Adverse reactions to food

Diana Vergnano

When we talk about adverse reactions to food (ARFs) we mean an abnormal response to one or more components of the food. ARFs can be classified in different ways; one of the most commonly used will be proposed here. According to this classification, ARFs are mainly divided into immune-mediated reactions (definable food allergies) and non-immune-mediated reactions (defined as food intolerances).

Immune-mediated reactions or food allergies

The pathophysiology of these reactions is not yet completely clear, but it is believed that there is an alteration in the normal enteric processing of antigens and in the development of oral tolerance. Commonly the antigens are proteins, which must have a minimum size to trigger the reaction. In human medicine it has been established that the minimum size is between 10 and 70 kD.

Immunoglobulins are synthesized after the first contact with the allergen, so the first time it is taken it is normally tolerated.

In this category we can mention:

- *IgE-mediated reactions (type I hypersensitivity)*. Among allergies, IgE-mediated allergies are thought to be the majority. These reactions can cause symptoms of immediate hypersensitivity (from a few minutes to hours after ingestion) and intermediate/delayed (from a few hours to a few days), the latter caused by the release of cytokines by mast cells activated by IgE;
- *reactions not mediated by IgE (type II, III, IV hypersensitivity)*. There is little information regarding this type of reactions, however it seems that type III and IV mechanisms (hypersensitivity mediated by immune complexes or cell-mediated) may be involved in dogs and cats, unlike the type II (cytotoxic reactions). These reactions give rise to symptoms of delayed hypersensitivity (from a few hours to a few days).

Non-immune-mediated reactions or food intolerances

The pathophysiology of food intolerances varies for each type of reaction. Even ingredients that do not contain proteins, such as some additives, are thought to trigger this type of reaction.

In this category there are recognized:

- *Idiosyncratic or idiopathic reactions*. This term indicates reactions that mimic an allergic reaction, but do not involve the immune system. They differ from allergies because they can also occur at the first contact with the responsible substance, but the triggering mechanism is unknown.
- *Food poisoning*. This are caused by the presence of a toxin in the food, usually of a bacterial or fungal origin. Some typical examples are myco-toxins and botulinum toxin.
- *Metabolic or enzymatic food reactions*. They are caused by a metabolic abnormality, such as an enzyme deficiency in the gastrointestinal tract. The typical example is lactose intolerance: since the enzyme is usually present, but in smaller quantities, the reaction is dose-dependent, unlike what is observed for food allergies.
- *Pharmacological reactions*. They are also dose dependent and, for example, they are observed when foods contain high dosages of vasoactive amines, such as histamine. The most typical case is the ingestion of deteriorated fish, in which histidine is decarboxylated to histamine by bacteria. The classic symptoms that mimic an allergic reaction occur, which include itching, erythema, vomiting and diarrhea.

Symptomatology

ARFs express mainly dermatological and/or gastroenteric symptoms, not necessarily in combination with each-other. Dermatological symptoms are highly variable, and the main ones include:

- non-seasonal itching, which can be generalized or localized;
- erythema, grazes, external otitis and dog pododermatitis;
- miliary dermatitis, eosinophilic plaques, self-induced symmetric alopecia in cats.

Gastrointestinal symptoms include diarrhea and sometimes vomiting and abdominal pain.

Diagnosis

There is currently no predisposition of age, gender or breed, although clinical signs often occur in very young animals. The combination of dermatological and gastroenteric symptoms strongly advocates the diagnosis of ARF.

The diagnosis is obtained by evaluating the response to diet therapy, that is, the elimination diet, after excluding other pathologies that could cause similar symptoms (for example parasitic dermatitis, flea allergy dermatitis, intestinal parasitosis).

Diet therapy: elimination diet

The goal of ARF nutritional management is to exclude from the diet the ingredient or ingredients that cause the patient's adverse reaction.

Since it is difficult to identify which component to avoid, the elimination diet system is adopted, which consists in administering a diet with ingredients to which the animal has never been exposed. The elimination diet is therefore at the same time a tool for diagnosis and therapy.

To set up an elimination diet, there are a few alternatives to choose from. There is absolutely no better option than the others, but the choice will have to depend on various factors, such as the species, the age and preferences of the patient, the type of management by the owner, the budget available. In addition, to make the best choice it is essential to obtain a nutritional history, or to draw up a list of all the foods that the animal has taken in its life. It is not only necessary to consider maintenance foods, but all that the animal may have ingested, including snacks, the owners' food and any drugs that contain flavoring or appetizing agents. The main alternatives are listed below.

Food based on new ingredients. The principle is based on the elimination of the ingredient which is guilty of having triggered the adverse reaction, introducing ingredients that have never been administered and to which, therefore, the animal's immune system has never been exposed.

Within this category there are two main options: using commercial foods or setting a homemade diet.

- *Commercial foods.* These are foods formulated with a single source of protein and/or a single source of carbohydrates, in the form of dry or wet foods (consisting of a single protein source, with or without a carbohydrate source). Many products of this type are available on the market, the so-called "monoproteins", and it is possible to choose between numerous and different protein sources. They have the advantage of being very practical for the owner and, in the case of dry foods and some wet foods, they have the advantage of being complete (to verify it, it is sufficient to evaluate whether the wording "complete food" or "complementary food" is present on the label, as it is mandatory by law). If it is a question of complementary food, it must be kept in mind that it can be used as the only food for limited periods and only if it is an adult animal; in other cases they must be suitably integrated.

- *Homemade diet.* Usually it is formulated by choosing a protein source and a source of carbohydrates (which also contains proteins) which are new for the animal (for example horse and potatoes). The main advantage is that of being able to safely exclude the presence of other protein sources or additives that could be responsible for ARFs. The disadvantages are the lack of practicality of this type of diet, which requires greater efforts from the owner, and they often have a higher cost. Furthermore, if the diet is formulated with only two ingredients, it will undoubtedly not be complete and consequently it can be used for short periods and integrated later. For this purpose, it will be advisable to choose special minerals and vitamin supplements, giving priority to those without flavorings or appetizers.

Foods based on hydrolyzed proteins. They are based on the concept that in order to trigger an immune reaction, a protein must have a certain size: if the protein is hydrolyzed, and therefore split into peptides with very small dimensions, it cannot give adverse reactions. There are various types of this type on the market; some combine hydrolyzed protein with an uncommon source of carbohydrates, others use purified starch. These diets can be a good option when it is difficult to identify a new protein source because the patient has already been exposed to many protein sources or because the nutritional history is incomplete. Furthermore, this choice has the advantage of being practical for the owner, albeit quite expensive.

Duration of the elimination diet

The elimination diet should be carried out for at least 8-12 weeks when dermatological symptoms are present and 2-4 weeks if there are only gastrointestinal symptoms.

It is very important that the elimination diet is carried out correctly by the owner and that the animal is kept under strict control during this period (for example the cat that normally has access to the outside must be kept indoors, the dog must always be kept on a leash when going out). If the animal ingests a food not present in the elimination diet, the test must be repeated from the beginning.

If the clinical symptoms do not improve and it is certain that the elimination diet has been carried out correctly by the owner, it is advisable to test a second elimination diet, different from the first, because there is a possibility that the chosen ingredients were not really new for the patient or that the patient experiences adverse reactions to more than one ingredient. In addition, there is the antigenic cross-reactivity, that is, the possibility that the animal reacts to different proteins but with similar amino acid sequences.

If clinical symptoms improve only partially, the possibility of other concomitant pathologies, such as atopic dermatitis and environmental allergies, should also be considered.

Challenge test

Animals that have clinically improved with the elimination diet should be given the ingredients of the previous diet again, to obtain a true diagnosis of ARF.

The introduction of a single ingredient at a time for 1-2 weeks should make it possible to identify which ingredient was responsible.

In practice, however, this system is difficult to apply: the owners often, having solved the problem, are not interested in carrying out the test, moreover it is not always easy to identify all the ingredients present in a commercial food and, lastly, it is not said that the test works because of the diversity of heat treatments and ingredient production processes; it seems that certain allergens, in fact, are deactivated or, on the contrary, are formed with high temperatures.

The reintroduction of the previous diet is certainly more easily practicable, even if it is not always obvious to have the owner's compliance; in this case the recurrence of the symptoms allows us to make a diagnosis of the ARF, but not to identify the responsible ingredient.

Retention

Once the ARF has been diagnosed, it will be necessary to choose an adequate maintenance food: if a complete food has been used for the diagnosis (hydrolyzed, complete monoprotein or a complete homemade diet), it will be possible to keep the same food; if a complementary food or an incomplete home diet has been used, the diet must be suitably balanced.

Some animals with ARFs may develop new adverse reactions over time; if this occurs, you will need to change the ingredients of the diet again.

Heart diseases

Heart diseases are common in dogs and even more so in cats. In recent years, medical therapy has improved and allows to increase the life expectancy and, above all, to maintain a good quality of life, controlling the clinical signs and the progression of these pathologies. There are several risk factors, which can cause or complicate these diseases, which must always be taken into consideration (Table 4.21). In this paragraph we will see what are the most important nutrients that generally concern heart diseases, specifying from time to time for which pathological process they may be most relevant.

One of the keys to success in the medical therapy of cardiac pathologies is nutrition, as it is able to help slow the progression of the disease, improve the quality of life and also reduce the number or doses of some drugs (especially diuretics). Usually these pathologies are followed by the specialist, but the control of the diet and of the patient, in general and over time, is certainly within our competence.

■ **TABLE 4.21 - RISK FACTORS FOR HEART DISEASES**

Breed
Sex
Obesity
Kidney disease
Drugs
Endocrinopathies
Heartworms

The first real big goal, common to the treatment of all pathologies and even more than cardiac ones, is to provide the correct amount of kcal avoiding excesses or deficiencies.

First of all, we need to evaluate BCS and MCS, as we have seen previously. As always, the owner's compliance is important and we must constantly investigate whether, what and how much the animal eats, if the owner follows our advice, if he provides treats, snacks etc. As in the case of CRF, in very advanced stages of the disease it is necessary to compromise on what it would be necessary to eat and what the animal would like to eat, to avoid deficiencies and above all to avoid or limit what is commonly called cardiac cachexia.

Cardiac cachexia is prevalent in animals with congestive heart failure (CHF) and appears to be linked to a multifactorial process that leads to anorexia, increased needs and production of inflammatory cytokines (e.g. tumor necrosis factor, interleukin 1), which exacerbate the process and also induce lean mass catabolism.

Although obesity is a predisposing factor for heart disease, obese animals are less predisposed and more protected from the effects of CHF. This is known as the "obesity paradox". In these animals the capricious appetite is typical, especially in the worsening phase. It has been seen that, just before a clinical worsening of the disease, especially in CHF, animals reduce the amount of food ingested or become anorexic. This can be useful in trying to prevent worsening, reevaluating them and making changes or adjustments to therapy if necessary.

For this reason, we must make sure that the owner is sensitized and quickly communicates any decrease in appetite to us.

The diet for a heart diseased animal is always a challenge. There is no ideal diet that is always valid, but the diet must be adapted to the type of pathology, the stage in which it is found, the animal and any concomitant pathologies, such as CRF. The nutrients to be taken into consideration are different, there are also some available studies that report some reference quantities (Table 4.22). The quantity of proteins must be adequate and their restriction is foreseen only in case of CRF; moreover, they must be of high quality and highly digestible.

■ **TABLE 4.22 - LEVELS OF NUTRITIONAL FACTORS TO CONSIDER IN THE FOOD IN THE DM**

Nutrients	Dogs	Cats
Sodium	0.15-0.25%, asymptomatic phase 0.08-0.15%, symptomatic phase	0.07-0.3%
Potassium	0.4%	0.52%
Magnesium	>0.06%	>0.04%
Taurine	0.1%	>0.3%
L-carnitine	0.02%	-

DM = dry matter.

Sodium

A minimal restriction of sodium is indicated in the early stages of heart disease, although there are no studies showing particular benefits regarding the delay of its progression (see Table 4.22). It is not indicated or even not recommended in the absence of symptoms, as sodium deficiency can activate or anticipate the activation of the renin-angiotensin-aldosterone system (RAAS), with the consequences that we know well.

When the symptoms and/or dilatation become evident, then a greater restriction is recommended (see Table 4.22), especially if diuretic drugs are used. All possible sources of sodium must be evaluated, from diet to treats, from snacks to water.

In the advanced stages, the use of distilled water or water containing a maximum of 150 ppm sodium can be considered. This element is obviously important in the course of CHF, but it is recommended to reduce it also in hypertensive animals, to better control the pressure, obviously in association with medical therapy, which remains the most effective therapy today (amlodipine). It is important to explain to the owner that, unlike humans, dogs and cats much more willingly accept a restriction of sodium in food and that any lack of appetite may be linked to other factors (often to drugs or to an imminent worsening of the disease).

Potassium and magnesium

These two elements must surely be monitored. Hyperkalaemia, hypokalaemia and hypomagnesaemia can also occur due to the effect of the drugs that are used, resulting in arrhythmias, alteration of contractility, greater side effects than cardiac drugs: shortly, a worsening of the general conditions. Obviously, the diet or the supplements will be chosen according to the present alteration (see Table 4.22), evaluating and checking from time to time the commercial diets that we have available or considering the use of a dedicated homemade diet.

Taurine

As we have seen, taurine is an essential amino acid in cats, but in the presence of a cardiac pathology it is absolutely recommended to integrate it also in dogs (see Table 4.22). Taurine has an action of osmoregulation and calcium-modulation, inactivates free radicals and is a natural antagonist of angiotensin II.

In cats, its deficiency is responsible for the dilated myocardiopathy; in dogs, there are some particularly predisposed breeds such as the Cocker Spaniel, Labrador Retriever, Dalmatian, English Bulldog etc. (Table 4.23). We therefore recommend its integration if there is only the suspicion of a deficiency, without certainty. Both in dogs and in cats, if given in excess it has no side effects.

L-carnitine

It is synthesized starting from lysine and methionine and is an essential component of the enzymes of the mitochondrial membrane, which transport the fatty acids used as energy; also, it has a detoxification action on the mitochondria.

In dogs, its deficiency is associated with dilated myocardiopathy. In general, it is secondary (see Table 4.23), but in the Boxer, as in humans, it can be primary. Its integration, especially in this breed, is recommended, although unfortunately we have to deal with the costs, which are often very high in cardiac therapy.

▦ **TABLE 4.23 - POSSIBLE CAUSES OF L-CARNITINE AND TAURINE DEFICIENCY IN DOGS**

Dogs fed with low protein levels	Carnitine and taurine
Vegetarian dogs	Carnitine and taurine

Antioxidants

Other nutrients that we can consider are omega-3 fatty acids (EPA, DHA), which are very useful as they reduce the formation of inflammatory cytokines and the loss of lean mass, especially during CHF, and have an anti-arrhythmic effect. The recommended dose is 40 mg/kg of EPA and 25 mg/kg of DHA per day.

Finally, antioxidants can play an important role in heart diseases thanks to their control over free radicals, especially those of oxygen, the so-called ROS (Reactive Oxygen Species), especially in dilated cardiomyopathy (DCM), in chronic valve disease (CVD) or in the progress of advanced CHF, when there is an increase in their production and the coverage of endogenous antioxidants may not be enough. Studies on this topic are not many and for now a dose of reference is still not available.

Chapter 5

The recipes

The watchword is "graduality"

OBJECTIVES OF THIS CHAPTER

- Choose the recipe for our patient/owner based on their needs
- Indicate precisely to the owner the quantities needed to cover the patient's needs

In this chapter we find some useful home recipes for adult dogs and cats. They are maintenance recipes for active and non-active, hypoallergenic animals, which have vegetarian or raw food diets. They offer a valid and rapid alternative to commercial diets and meet the needs of the animal and the owner. They cannot be exhaustive or replace a dedicated nutritional plan, but they can be useful in the short term, together with the application of the knowledge acquired so far.

Some advice for the owner: the meat and fish can be steamed, grilled or cooked with a little water. The meat can also be given raw, but only that of bovine and after having frozen it for at least 48 hours. Internal organs such as heart, kidneys, lungs, spleen can also be used; it is recommended to use the liver in small quantities.

As we have seen, we can use as a source of carbohydrates pasta, Baby pasta, couscous etc., normal or wholemeal (especially if we want to increase the fiber quota), or gluten-free foods such as potatoes, polenta, rice, quinoa, tapioca etc.

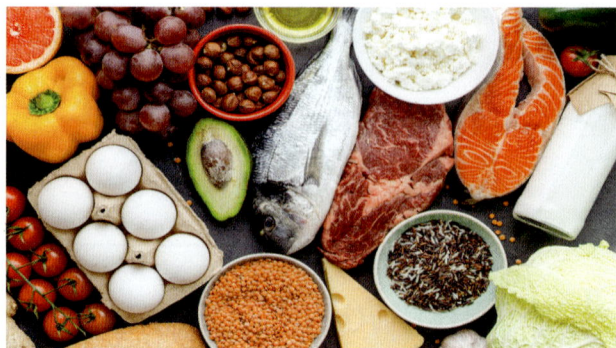

■ **FIGURE 5.1** A balanced diet must be based on a variety of healthy foods.

Pasta, rice etc. must be cooked but not "overcooked" (it is better to cook them for a few minutes longer than the time indicated on the package) and it is not necessary to rinse them after cooking.

Among the vegetables you can use are carrots, squash, green beans, courgettes and leafy vegetables such as chard, chicory, spinach, lettuce etc. The amount of vegetables can be increased or decreased according to the consistency of the stool and it is more appropriate that they are cooked, mashed or blended.

Fruits, such as apples, pears and peaches, should be given primarily as a treat. Fruits that contain a lot of fructose (e.g. banana, melon, watermelon) should be given with caution. It is important to know that fruits also affect stool consistency.

The fats to be used are sunflower and corn oil, but also, alternatively, olive oil, salmon, butter and lard oil. It is very important not to replace the ingredients in the recipes with others or to eliminate some of them. All the ingredients must be mixed so that the animal cannot choose some of them over others (Figure 5.1).

The indicated diet should be given daily and must be divided into the different meals. The weight of the ingredients is considered raw. You can also choose between two supplements to balance the recipes.

The diet must be introduced gradually over a period of 1 week to 10 days, preferably one new ingredient at a time. The weight indicated in the diets corresponds to the animal that is in perfect shape, that is, with a BCS of 5/9. If the animal is overweight or underweight, we will have to choose a diet that indicates the weight we want our patient to reach.

Maintenance recipes for the active adult dog

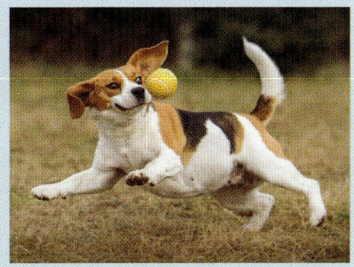

 **Weight:** 5 kg
kcal: around 370

1

Ingredients	Quantity
Chicken breast/Turkey	100 g
Rice/Pasta	50 g
Sunflower/Corn oil	2 teaspoons
Vegetables (carrot, pumpkin, courgette, green beans, chard, spinach, chicory, lettuce etc.)	60 g
Bread	20 g
Supplements	*

* Completa Q Diet/Trovet Balance (3 g) or Essential Adult (5 g)

2

Ingredients	Quantity
Hake/Cod	140 g
Rice/Pasta	50 g
Sunflower oil	2 teaspoons
Vegetables (carrot, pumpkin, courgette, green beans, chard, spinach, chicory, lettuce etc.)	60 g
Bread	20 g
Supplements	*

* Completa Q Diet/Trovet Balance (3 g) or Essential Adult (5 g)

3

Ingredients	Quantity
Lean beef/Pork rump	100 g
Rice/Pasta	30 g
Sunflower/Corn oil	2 teaspoons
Vegetables (carrot, pumpkin, courgette, green beans, chard, spinach, chicory, lettuce etc.)	60 g
Bread	20 g
Supplements	*

* Completa Q Diet/Trovet Balance (3 g) or Essential Adult (5 g)

 **Weight:** 10 kg
kcal: around 600

1

Ingredients	Quantity
Chicken breast/Turkey	200 g
Rice/Pasta	60 g
Sunflower/Corn oil	4 teaspoons
Vegetables (carrot, pumpkin, courgette, green beans, chard, spinach, chicory, lettuce etc.)	60 g
Bread	40 g
Supplements	*

* Completa Q Diet/Trovet Balance (5 g) or Essential Adult (7 g)

2

Ingredients	Quantity
Hake/Cod	220 g
Rice/Pasta	80 g
Sunflower oil	4 teaspoons
Vegetables (carrot, pumpkin, courgette, green beans, chard, spinach, chicory, lettuce etc.)	60 g
Bread	40 g
Supplements	*

* Completa Q Diet/Trovet Balance (5 g) or Essential Adult (7 g)

3

Ingredients	Quantity
Lean beef/Pork rump	180 g
Rice/Pasta	40 g
Sunflower/Corn oil	4 teaspoons
Vegetables (carrot, pumpkin, courgette, green beans, chard, spinach, chicory, lettuce etc.)	60 g
Bread	40 g
Supplements	*

* Completa Q Diet/Trovet Balance (5 g) or Essential Adult (7 g)

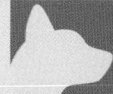

Weight: 15 kg
kcal: around 840

1

Ingredients	Quantity
Chicken breast/Turkey	200 g
Rice/Pasta	60 g
Sunflower/Corn oil	6 teaspoons
Vegetables (carrot, pumpkin, courgette, green beans, chard, spinach, chicory, lettuce etc.)	60 g
Bread	100 g
Supplements	*

* Completa Q Diet/Trovet Balance (6 g) or Essential Adult (9 g)

2

Ingredients	Quantity
Hake/Cod	240 g
Rice/Pasta	70 g
Sunflower oil	6 teaspoons
Vegetables (carrot, pumpkin, courgette, green beans, chard, spinach, chicory, lettuce etc.)	60 g
Bread	100 g
Supplements	*

* Completa Q Diet/Trovet Balance (6 g) or Essential Adult (9 g)

3

Ingredients	Quantity
Lean beef/Pork rump	180 g
Rice/Pasta	50 g
Sunflower/Corn oil	6 teaspoons
Vegetables (carrot, pumpkin, courgette, green beans, chard, spinach, chicory, lettuce etc.)	60 g
Bread	100 g
Supplements	*

* Completa Q Diet/Trovet Balance (6 g) or Essential Adult (9 g)

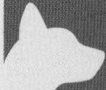

Weight: 20 kg
kcal: around 1,000

1

Ingredients	Quantity
Chicken breast/Turkey	300 g
Rice/Pasta	80 g
Sunflower/Corn oil	6 teaspoons
Vegetables (carrot, pumpkin, courgette, green beans, chard, spinach, chicory, lettuce etc.)	60 g
Bread	100 g
Supplements	*

* Completa Q Diet/Trovet Balance (8 g) or Essential Adult (11 g)

2

Ingredients	Quantity
Hake/Cod	350 g
Rice/Pasta	90 g
Sunflower oil	6 teaspoons
Vegetables (carrot, pumpkin, courgette, green beans, chard, spinach, chicory, lettuce etc.)	60 g
Bread	100 g
Supplements	*

* Completa Q Diet/Trovet Balance (8 g) or Essential Adult (11 g)

2

Ingredients	Quantity
Lean beef/Pork rump	250 g
Rice/Pasta	60 g
Sunflower/Corn oil	6 teaspoons
Vegetables (carrot, pumpkin, courgette, green beans, chard, spinach, chicory, lettuce etc.)	60 g
Bread	100 g
Supplements	*

* Completa Q Diet/Trovet Balance (8 g) or Essential Adult (11 g)

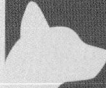

Weight: 30 kg
kcal: around 1,400

1

Ingredients	Quantity
Chicken breast/Turkey	500 g
Rice/Pasta	130 g
Sunflower/Corn oil	8 teaspoons
Vegetables (carrot, pumpkin, courgette, green beans, chard, spinach, chicory, lettuce etc.)	100 g
Bread	100 g
Supplements	*

* Completa Q Diet/Trovet Balance (10 g) or Essential Adult (14 g)

2

Ingredients	Quantity
Hake/Cod	600 g
Rice/Pasta	160 g
Sunflower oil	8 teaspoons
Vegetables (carrot, pumpkin, courgette, green beans, chard, spinach, chicory, lettuce etc.)	100 g
Bread	100 g
Supplements	*

* Completa Q Diet/Trovet Balance (10 g) or Essential Adult (14 g)

3

Ingredients	Quantity
Lean beef/Pork rump	450 g
Rice/Pasta	80 g
Sunflower/Corn oil	8 teaspoons
Vegetables (carrot, pumpkin, courgette, green beans, chard, spinach, chicory, lettuce etc.)	100 g
Bread	100 g
Supplements	*

* Completa Q Diet/Trovet Balance (10 g) or Essential Adult (14 g)

Light maintenance recipes for the underactive, sterilized/neutered adult dog

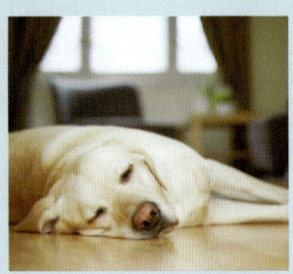

Weight: 5 kg
kcal: around 290

1

Ingredients	Quantity
Chicken breast/Turkey	130 g
Rice/Pasta	20 g
Sunflower/Corn oil	1 teaspoon
Vegetables (carrot, pumpkin, courgette, green beans, chard, spinach, chicory, lettuce etc.)	60 g
Bread	20 g
Supplements	*

* Completa Q Diet/Trovet Balance (3 g) or Essential Adult (5 g)

2

Ingredients	Quantity
Hake/Cod	160 g
Rice/Pasta	30 g
Sunflower oil	1 teaspoon
Vegetables (carrot, pumpkin, courgette, green beans, chard, spinach, chicory, lettuce etc.)	60 g
Bread	20 g
Supplements	*

* Completa Q Diet/Trovet Balance (3 g) or Essential Adult (5 g)

3

Ingredients	Quantity
Lean beef/Pork rump	110 g
Rice/Pasta	10 g
Sunflower/Corn oil	1 teaspoon
Vegetables (carrot, pumpkin, courgette, green beans, chard, spinach, chicory, lettuce etc.)	60 g
Bread	20 g
Supplements	*

* Completa Q Diet/Trovet Balance (3 g) or Essential Adult (5 g)

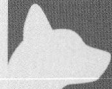

Weight: 10 kg
kcal: around 480

1

Ingredients	Quantity
Chicken breast/Turkey	180 g
Rice/Pasta	40 g
Sunflower/Corn oil	4 teaspoons
Vegetables (carrot, pumpkin, courgette, green beans, chard, spinach, chicory, lettuce etc.)	60 g
Bread	20 g
Supplements	*

* Completa Q Diet/Trovet Balance (5 g) or Essential Adult (7 g)

2

Ingredients	Quantity
Hake/Cod	260 g
Rice/Pasta	40 g
Sunflower oil	4 teaspoons
Vegetables (carrot, pumpkin, courgette, green beans, chard, spinach, chicory, lettuce etc.)	60 g
Bread	20 g
Supplements	*

* Completa Q Diet/Trovet Balance (5 g) or Essential Adult (7 g)

3

Ingredients	Quantity
Lean beef/Pork rump	190 g
Rice/Pasta	20 g
Sunflower/Corn oil	2 teaspoons
Vegetables (carrot, pumpkin, courgette, green beans, chard, spinach, chicory, lettuce etc.)	60 g
Bread	20 g
Supplements	*

* Completa Q Diet/Trovet Balance (5 g) or Essential Adult (7 g)

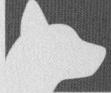 **Weight:** 15 kg
kcal: around 670

1

Ingredients	Quantity
Chicken breast/Turkey	220 g
Rice/Pasta	40 g
Sunflower/Corn oil	6 teaspoons
Vegetables (carrot, pumpkin, courgette, green beans, chard, spinach, chicory, lettuce etc.)	60 g
Bread	50 g
Supplements	*

* Completa Q Diet/Trovet Balance (6 g) or Essential Adult (9 g)

2

Ingredients	Quantity
Hake/Cod	260 g
Rice/Pasta	60 g
Sunflower oil	6 teaspoons
Vegetables (carrot, pumpkin, courgette, green beans, chard, spinach, chicory, lettuce etc.)	60 g
Bread	50 g
Supplements	*

* Completa Q Diet/Trovet Balance (6 g) or Essential Adult (9 g)

3

Ingredients	Quantity
Lean beef/Pork rump	220 g
Rice/Pasta	30 g
Sunflower/Corn oil	4 teaspoons
Vegetables (carrot, pumpkin, courgette, green beans, chard, spinach, chicory, lettuce etc.)	60 g
Bread	50 g
Supplements	*

* Completa Q Diet/Trovet Balance (6 g) or Essential Adult (9 g)

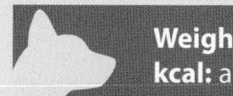

Weight: 20 kg
kcal: around 800

1

Ingredients	Quantity
Chicken breast/Turkey	330 g
Rice/Pasta	60 g
Sunflower/Corn oil	6 teaspoons
Vegetables (carrot, pumpkin, courgette, green beans, chard, spinach, chicory, lettuce etc.)	60 g
Bread	50 g
Supplements	*

* Completa Q Diet/Trovet Balance (8 g) or Essential Adult (11 g)

2

Ingredients	Quantity
Hake/Cod	380 g
Rice/Pasta	80 g
Sunflower oil	6 teaspoons
Vegetables (carrot, pumpkin, courgette, green beans, chard, spinach, chicory, lettuce etc.)	60 g
Bread	50 g
Supplements	*

* Completa Q Diet/Trovet Balance (8 g) or Essential Adult (11 g)

3

Ingredients	Quantity
Lean beef/Pork rump	300 g
Rice/Pasta	40 g
Sunflower/Corn oil	4 teaspoons
Vegetables (carrot, pumpkin, courgette, green beans, chard, spinach, chicory, lettuce etc.)	60 g
Bread	50 g
Supplements	*

* Completa Q Diet/Trovet Balance (8 g) or Essential Adult (11 g)

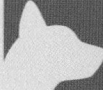

Weight: 30 kg
kcal: around 1,100

1

Ingredients	Quantity
Chicken breast/Turkey	450 g
Rice/Pasta	100 g
Sunflower/Corn oil	6 teaspoons
Vegetables (carrot, pumpkin, courgette, green beans, chard, spinach, chicory, lettuce etc.)	100 g
Bread	50 g
Supplements	*

* Completa Q Diet/Trovet Balance (10 g) or Essential Adult (14 g)

2

Ingredients	Quantity
Hake/Cod	600 g
Rice/Pasta	110 g
Sunflower oil	6 teaspoons
Vegetables (carrot, pumpkin, courgette, green beans, chard, spinach, chicory, lettuce etc.)	100 g
Bread	50 g
Supplements	*

* Completa Q Diet/Trovet Balance (10 g) or Essential Adult (14 g)

3

Ingredients	Quantity
Lean beef/Pork rump	450 g
Rice/Pasta	50 g
Sunflower/Corn oil	6 teaspoons
Vegetables (carrot, pumpkin, courgette, green beans, chard, spinach, chicory, lettuce etc.)	100 g
Bread	50 g
Supplements	*

* Completa Q Diet/Trovet Balance (10 g) or Essential Adult (14 g)

Maintenance recipes for active (hypoallergenic) and underactive, sterilized/neutered (hypoallergenic light) adult dogs

The recipes are complete and balanced, but it is recommended to give only meat, carbohydrates and oil for the first 45 days-2 months (the time it takes to make the diagnosis) and to integrate them only later.

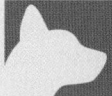

Weight: 5 kg
kcal: around 370

Ingredients	Quantity
Lean rabbit meat	80 g
Tapioca	50 g
Sunflower oil	2 teaspoons
Vegetables (pumpkin)	60 g
Supplements	*

Not to be administered in the period of diagnosis

* Completa Q Diet/Trovet Balance (3 g) or Essential Adult (5 g)

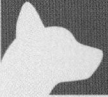

Weight: 5 kg
kcal: around 290 (light)

Ingredients	Quantity
Lean rabbit meat	60 g
Tapioca	40 g
Sunflower oil	1 teaspoon
Vegetables (pumpkin)	60 g
Supplements	*

Not to be administered in the period of diagnosis

* Completa Q Diet/Trovet Balance (3 g) or Essential Adult (5 g)

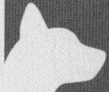 **Weight:** 10 kg
kcal: around 600

Ingredients	Quantity
Lean rabbit meat	120 g
Tapioca	80 g
Sunflower oil	4 teaspoons
Vegetables (pumpkin)	60 g
Supplements	*

Not to be administered
in the period of diagnosis

* Completa Q Diet/Trovet Balance (5 g) or Essential Adult (7 g)

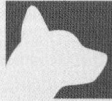 **Weight:** 10 kg
kcal: around 480 (light)

Ingredients	Quantity
Lean rabbit meat	100 g
Tapioca	60 g
Sunflower oil	4 teaspoons
Vegetables (pumpkin)	60 g
Supplements	*

Not to be administered
in the period of diagnosis

* Completa Q Diet/Trovet Balance (5 g) or Essential Adult (7 g)

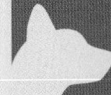

Weight: 15 kg
kcal: around 840

Ingredients	Quantity
Lean rabbit meat	160 g
Tapioca	110 g
Sunflower oil	6 teaspoons
Vegetables (pumpkin)	60 g
Supplements	*

Not to be administered
in the period of diagnosis

* Completa Q Diet/Trovet Balance (6 g) or Essential Adult (9 g)

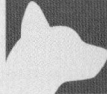

Weight: 15 kg
kcal: around 670 (light)

Ingredients	Quantity
Lean rabbit meat	140 g
Tapioca	80 g
Sunflower oil	6 teaspoons
Vegetables (pumpkin)	60 g
Supplements	*

Not to be administered
in the period of diagnosis

* Completa Q Diet/Trovet Balance (6 g) or Essential Adult (9 g)

Weight: 20 kg
kcal: around 1,000

Ingredients	Quantity
Lean rabbit meat	210 g
Tapioca	130 g
Sunflower oil	6 teaspoons
Vegetables (pumpkin)	100 g
Supplements	*

Not to be administered in the period of diagnosis

* Completa Q Diet/Trovet Balance (8 g) or Essential Adult (11 g)

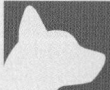

Weight: 20 kg
kcal: around 800 (light)

Ingredients	Quantity
Lean rabbit meat	170 g
Tapioca	120 g
Sunflower oil	4 teaspoons
Vegetables (pumpkin)	60 g
Supplements	*

Not to be administered in the period of diagnosis

* Completa Q Diet/Trovet Balance (8 g) or Essential Adult (11 g)

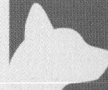

Weight: 30 kg
kcal: around 1,400

Ingredients	Quantity
Lean rabbit meat	300 g
Tapioca	200 g
Sunflower oil	8 teaspoons
Vegetables (pumpkin)	100 g
Supplements	*

Not to be administered
in the period of diagnosis

* Completa Q Diet/Trovet Balance (10 g) or Essential Adult (14 g)

Weight: 30 kg
kcal: around 1,100 (light)

Ingredients	Quantity
Lean rabbit meat	250 g
Tapioca	150 g
Sunflower oil	4 teaspoons
Vegetables (pumpkin)	100 g
Supplements	*

Not to be administered
in the period of diagnosis

* Completa Q Diet/Trovet Balance (10 g) or Essential Adult (14 g)

Maintenance recipes for active (grain-free) and underactive, sterilized/neutered (grain-free light) adult dogs

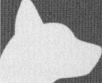

Weight: 5 kg
kcal: around 370

Ingredients	Quantity
Pork loin	100 g
Peeled potatoes	150 g
Sunflower oil	2 teaspoons
Vegetables (carrot, pumpkin, courgette, green beans, chard, spinach, chicory, lettuce etc.)	60 g
Apple	50 g
Supplements	*

* Completa Q Diet/Trovet Balance (3 g) or Essential Adult (5 g)

Weight: 5 kg
kcal: around 290 (light)

Ingredients	Quantity
Pork loin	100 g
Peeled potatoes	70 g
Sunflower oil	1 teaspoon
Vegetables (carrot, pumpkin, courgette, green beans, chard, spinach, chicory, lettuce etc.)	60 g
Apple	50 g
Supplements	*

* Completa Q Diet/Trovet Balance (3 g) or Essential Adult (5 g)

Weight: 10 kg
kcal: around 600

Ingredients	Quantity
Pork loin	200 g
Peeled potatoes	280 g
Sunflower oil	2 teaspoons
Vegetables (carrot, pumpkin, courgette, green beans, chard, spinach, chicory, lettuce etc.)	60 g
Apple	50 g
Supplements	*

* Completa Q Diet/Trovet Balance (5 g) or Essential Adult (7 g)

Weight: 10 kg
kcal: around 480 (light)

Ingredients	Quantity
Pork loin	200 g
Peeled potatoes	170 g
Sunflower oil	1 teaspoon
Vegetables (carrot, pumpkin, courgette, green beans, chard, spinach, chicory, lettuce etc.)	60 g
Apple	50 g
Supplements	*

* Completa Q Diet/Trovet Balance (5 g) or Essential Adult (7 g)

Weight: 15 kg
kcal: around 840

Ingredients	Quantity
Pork loin	250 g
Peeled potatoes	400 g
Sunflower oil	4 teaspoons
Vegetables (carrot, pumpkin, courgette, green beans, chard, spinach, chicory, lettuce etc.)	60 g
Apple	100 g
Supplements	*

* Completa Q Diet/Trovet Balance (6 g) or Essential Adult (9 g)

Weight: 15 kg
kcal: around 670 (light)

Ingredients	Quantity
Pork loin	250 g
Peeled potatoes	260 g
Sunflower oil	2 teaspoons
Vegetables (carrot, pumpkin, courgette, green beans, chard, spinach, chicory, lettuce etc.)	60 g
Apple	100 g
Supplements	*

* Completa Q Diet/Trovet Balance (6 g) or Essential Adult (9 g)

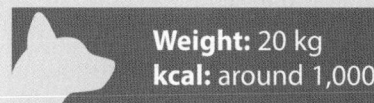

Weight: 20 kg
kcal: around 1,000

Ingredients	Quantity
Pork loin	350 g
Peeled potatoes	450 g
Sunflower oil	4 teaspoons
Vegetables (carrot, pumpkin, courgette, green beans, chard, spinach, chicory, lettuce etc.)	60 g
Apple	100 g
Supplements	*

* Completa Q Diet/Trovet Balance (8 g) or Essential Adult (11 g)

Weight: 20 kg
kcal: around 800 (light)

Ingredients	Quantity
Pork loin	350 g
Peeled potatoes	260 g
Sunflower oil	2 teaspoons
Vegetables (carrot, pumpkin, courgette, green beans, chard, spinach, chicory, lettuce etc.)	60 g
Apple	100 g
Supplements	*

* Completa Q Diet/Trovet Balance (8 g) or Essential Adult (11 g)

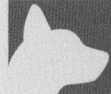

Weight: 30 kg
kcal: around 1,400

Ingredients	Quantity
Pork loin	500 g
Peeled potatoes	550 g
Sunflower oil	6 teaspoons
Vegetables (carrot, pumpkin, courgette, green beans, chard, spinach, chicory, lettuce etc.)	60 g
Apple	150 g
Supplements	*

* Completa Q Diet/Trovet Balance (10 g) or Essential Adult (14 g)

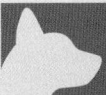

Weight: 30 kg
kcal: around 1,100 (light)

Ingredients	Quantity
Pork loin	500 g
Peeled potatoes	260 g
Sunflower oil	4 teaspoons
Vegetables (carrot, pumpkin, courgette, green beans, chard, spinach, chicory, lettuce etc.)	60 g
Apple	150 g
Supplements	*

* Completa Q Diet/Trovet Balance (10 g) or Essential Adult (14 g)

Maintenance recipes for active (BARF) and underactive, sterilized/neutered (BARF light) adult dogs

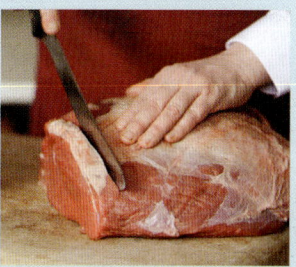

 **Weight:** 5 kg
kcal: around 370

Ingredients	Quantity
Beef without visible fat	70 g
Heart, spleen, kidneys, lungs, liver	30 g
Peeled potatoes	200 g
Sunflower oil	2 teaspoons
Vegetables (carrot, pumpkin, courgette, green beans, chard, spinach, chicory, lettuce etc.)	60 g
Apple	50 g
Supplements	*

* Completa Q Diet/Trovet Balance (3 g) or Essential Adult (5 g)

 **Weight:** 5 kg
kcal: around 290 (light)

Ingredients	Quantity
Beef without visible fat	70 g
Heart, spleen, kidneys, lungs, liver	30 g
Peeled potatoes	90 g
Sunflower oil	2 teaspoons
Vegetables (carrot, pumpkin, courgette, green beans, chard, spinach, chicory, lettuce etc.)	60 g
Apple	50 g
Supplements	*

* Completa Q Diet/Trovet Balance (3 g) or Essential Adult (5 g)

Weight: 10 kg
kcal: around 600

Ingredients	Quantity
Beef without visible fat	150 g
Heart, spleen, kidneys, lungs, liver	50 g
Peeled potatoes	280 g
Sunflower oil	2 teaspoons
Vegetables (carrot, pumpkin, courgette, green beans, chard, spinach, chicory, lettuce etc.)	60 g
Apple	50 g
Supplements	*

* Completa Q Diet/Trovet Balance (5 g) or Essential Adult (7 g)

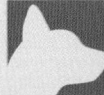

Weight: 10 kg
kcal: around 480 (light)

Ingredients	Quantity
Beef without visible fat	150 g
Heart, spleen, kidneys, lungs, liver	50 g
Peeled potatoes	170 g
Sunflower oil	1 teaspoon
Vegetables (carrot, pumpkin, courgette, green beans, chard, spinach, chicory, lettuce etc.)	60 g
Apple	50 g
Supplements	*

* Completa Q Diet/Trovet Balance (5 g) or Essential Adult (7 g)

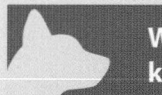

Weight: 15 kg
kcal: around 840

Ingredients	Quantity
Beef without visible fat	250 g
Heart, spleen, kidneys, lungs, liver	50 g
Peeled potatoes	400 g
Sunflower oil	4 teaspoons
Vegetables (carrot, pumpkin, courgette, green beans, chard, spinach, chicory, lettuce etc.)	60 g
Apple	50 g
Supplements	*

* Completa Q Diet/Trovet Balance (6 g) or Essential Adult (9 g)

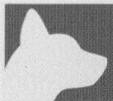

Weight: 15 kg
kcal: around 670 (light)

Ingredients	Quantity
Beef without visible fat	250 g
Heart, spleen, kidneys, lungs, liver	50 g
Peeled potatoes	200 g
Sunflower oil	2 teaspoons
Vegetables (carrot, pumpkin, courgette, green beans, chard, spinach, chicory, lettuce etc.)	60 g
Apple	100 g
Supplements	*

* Completa Q Diet/Trovet Balance (6 g) or Essential Adult (9 g)

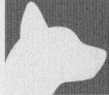

Weight: 20 kg
kcal: around 1,000

Ingredients	Quantity
Beef without visible fat	250 g
Heart, spleen, kidneys, lungs, liver	100 g
Peeled potatoes	460 g
Sunflower oil	4 teaspoons
Vegetables (carrot, pumpkin, courgette, green beans, chard, spinach, chicory, lettuce etc.)	60 g
Apple	100 g
Supplements	*

* Completa Q Diet/Trovet Balance (8 g) or Essential Adult (11 g)

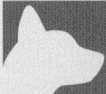

Weight: 20 kg
kcal: around 800 (light)

Ingredients	Quantity
Beef without visible fat	250 g
Heart, spleen, kidneys, lungs, liver	100 g
Peeled potatoes	280 g
Sunflower oil	2 teaspoons
Vegetables (carrot, pumpkin, courgette, green beans, chard, spinach, chicory, lettuce etc.)	60 g
Apple	100 g
Supplements	*

* Completa Q Diet/Trovet Balance (8 g) or Essential Adult (11 g)

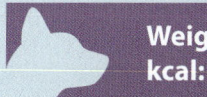

Weight: 30 kg
kcal: around 1,400

Ingredients	Quantity
Beef without visible fat	350 g
Heart, spleen, kidneys, lungs, liver	150 g
Peeled potatoes	600 g
Sunflower oil	6 teaspoons
Vegetables (carrot, pumpkin, courgette, green beans, chard, spinach, chicory, lettuce etc.)	60 g
Apple	150 g
Supplements	*

* Completa Q Diet/Trovet Balance (10 g) or Essential Adult (14 g)

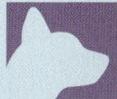

Weight: 30 kg
kcal: around 1,100 (light)

Ingredients	Quantity
Beef without visible fat	350 g
Heart, spleen, kidneys, lungs, liver	150 g
Peeled potatoes	300 g
Sunflower oil	4 teaspoons
Vegetables (carrot, pumpkin, courgette, green beans, chard, spinach, chicory, lettuce etc.)	60 g
Apple	150 g
Supplements	*

* Completa Q Diet/Trovet Balance (10 g) or Essential Adult (14 g)

Maintenance recipes for active (vegetarian) and underactive, sterilized/ neutered adult dogs (light vegetarian)

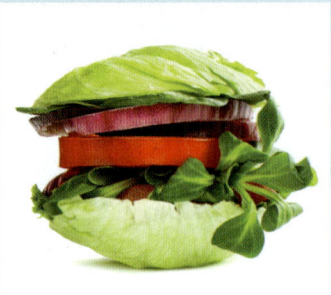

Weight: 5 kg
kcal: around 370

Ingredients	Quantity
Medium chicken egg	53 g (1 egg)
Chicken egg whites	74 g (2 egg whites)
Couscous	50 g
Sunflower oil	2 teaspoons
Vegetables (carrot, pumpkin, courgette, green beans, chard, spinach, chicory, lettuce etc.)	30 g
Low-fat plain yogurt	125 g
Supplements	*

* Completa Q Diet/Trovet Balance (3 g) or Essential Adult (5 g)

Weight: 5 kg
kcal: around 290 (light)

Ingredients	Quantity
Medium chicken egg	53 g (1 egg)
Chicken egg whites	74 g (2 egg whites)
Couscous	35 g
Sunflower oil	1 teaspoon
Vegetables (carrot, pumpkin, courgette, green beans, chard, spinach, chicory, lettuce etc.)	30 g
Low-fat plain yogurt	125 g
Supplements	*

* Completa Q Diet/Trovet Balance (3 g) or Essential Adult (5 g)

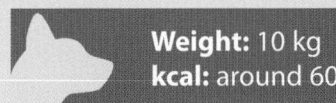

Weight: 10 kg
kcal: around 600

Ingredients	Quantity
Medium chicken egg	53 g (1 egg)
Chicken egg whites	185 g (5 egg whites)
Couscous	90 g
Sunflower oil	4 teaspoons
Vegetables (carrot, pumpkin, courgette, green beans, chard, spinach, chicory, lettuce etc.)	30 g
Low-fat plain yogurt	125 g
Supplements	*

* Completa Q Diet/Trovet Balance (5 g) or Essential Adult (7 g)

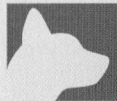

Weight: 10 kg
kcal: around 480 (light)

Ingredients	Quantity
Medium chicken egg	53 g (1 egg)
Chicken egg whites	185 g (5 egg whites)
Couscous	65 g
Sunflower oil	2 teaspoons
Vegetables (carrot, pumpkin, courgette, green beans, chard, spinach, chicory, lettuce etc.)	30 g
Low-fat plain yogurt	125 g
Supplements	*

* Completa Q Diet/Trovet Balance (5 g) or Essential Adult (7 g)

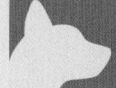

Weight: 15 kg
kcal: around 840

Ingredients	Quantity
Medium chicken egg	53 g (1 egg)
Chicken egg whites	259 g (7 egg whites)
Couscous	110 g
Sunflower oil	6 teaspoons
Grana cheese	20 g
Vegetables (carrot, pumpkin, courgette, green beans, chard, spinach, chicory, lettuce etc.)	60 g
Low-fat plain yogurt	125 g
Supplements	*

* Completa Q Diet/Trovet Balance (6 g) or Essential Adult (9 g)

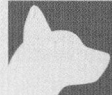

Weight: 15 kg
kcal: around 670 (light)

Ingredients	Quantity
Medium chicken egg	53 g (1 egg)
Chicken egg whites	259 g (7 egg whites)
Couscous	80 g
Sunflower oil	4 teaspoons
Grana cheese	20 g
Vegetables (carrot, pumpkin, courgette, green beans, chard, spinach, chicory, lettuce etc.)	60 g
Low-fat plain yogurt	125 g
Supplements	*

* Completa Q Diet/Trovet Balance (6 g) or Essential Adult (9 g)

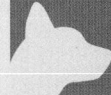

Weight: 20 kg
kcal: around 1,000

Ingredients	Quantity
Medium chicken egg	53 g (1 egg)
Chicken egg whites	259 g (7 egg whites)
Couscous	135 g
Sunflower oil	8 teaspoons
Grana cheese	30 g
Vegetables (carrot, pumpkin, courgette, green beans, chard, spinach, chicory, lettuce etc.)	60 g
Low-fat plain yogurt	125 g
Supplements	*

* Completa Q Diet/Trovet Balance (8 g) or Essential Adult (11 g)

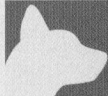

Weight: 20 kg
kcal: around 800 (light)

Ingredients	Quantity
Medium chicken egg	53 g (1 egg)
Chicken egg whites	259 g (7 egg whites)
Couscous	90 g
Sunflower oil	6 teaspoons
Grana cheese	30 g
Vegetables (carrot, pumpkin, courgette, green beans, chard, spinach, chicory, lettuce etc.)	60 g
Low-fat plain yogurt	125 g
Supplements	*

* Completa Q Diet/Trovet Balance (8 g) or Essential Adult (11 g)

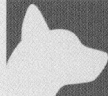

Weight: 30 kg
kcal: around 1,400

Ingredients	Quantity
Medium chicken egg	53 g (1 egg)
Chicken egg whites	296 g (8 egg whites)
Couscous	200 g
Sunflower oil	8 teaspoons
Grana cheese	70 g
Vegetables (carrot, pumpkin, courgette, green beans, chard, spinach, chicory, lettuce etc.)	100 g
Low-fat plain yogurt	125 g
Supplements	*

* Completa Q Diet/Trovet Balance (10 g) or Essential Adult (14 g)

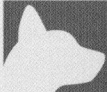

Weight: 30 kg
kcal: around 1,100 (light)

Ingredients	Quantity
Medium chicken egg	53 g (1 egg)
Chicken egg whites	296 g (8 egg whites)
Couscous	125 g
Sunflower oil	6 teaspoons
Grana cheese	70 g
Vegetables (carrot, pumpkin, courgette, green beans, chard, spinach, chicory, lettuce etc.)	100 g
Low-fat plain yogurt	125 g
Supplements	*

* Completa Q Diet/Trovet Balance (10 g) or Essential Adult (14 g)

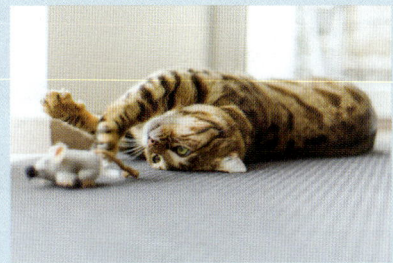

Maintenance recipes for the active adult cat

Weight: 3 kg
kcal: around 160

1

Ingredients	Quantity
Chicken breast	40 g
Chicken/Heart giblets, beef/pork spleen	50 g
Sunflower oil	1 teaspoon
Vegetables (pumpkin, carrot, courgette)	10 g
Supplements	*

* Completa Q Diet/Trovet Balance (2 g) or Essential Cat (2 g)

2

Ingredients	Quantity
Cod/Hake	110 g
Chicken/Heart giblets, beef/pork spleen	40 g
Sunflower oil	1 teaspoon
Vegetables (pumpkin, carrot, courgette)	10 g
Supplements	*

* Completa Q Diet/Trovet Balance (2 g) or Essential Cat (2 g)

Weight: 5 kg
kcal: around 234

1

Ingredients	Quantity
Chicken breast	100 g
Chicken/Heart giblets, beef/pork spleen	50 g
Sunflower oil	1 teaspoon
Vegetables (pumpkin, carrot, courgette)	20 g
Rice/Couscous/Pastina	5 g
Supplements	*

* Completa Q Diet/Trovet Balance (3 g) or Essential Cat (3 g)

2

Ingredients	Quantity
Cod/Hake	150 g
Chicken/Heart giblets, beef/pork spleen	50 g
Sunflower oil	2 teaspoons
Vegetables (pumpkin, carrot, courgette)	20 g
Rice/Couscous/Pastina	5 g
Supplements	*

* Completa Q Diet/Trovet Balance (3 g) or Essential Cat (3 g)

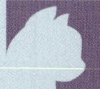

Weight: 8 kg
kcal: around 330

1

Ingredients	Quantity
Chicken breast	150 g
Chicken/Heart giblets, beef/pork spleen	50 g
Sunflower oil	2 teaspoons
Vegetables (pumpkin, carrot, courgette)	20 g
Rice/Couscous/Pastina	5 g
Supplements	*

* Completa Q Diet/Trovet Balance (3 g) or Essential Cat (3 g)

2

Ingredients	Quantity
Cod/Hake	160 g
Chicken/Heart giblets, beef/pork spleen	50 g
Sunflower oil	3 teaspoons
Vegetables (pumpkin, carrot, courgette)	20 g
Rice/Couscous/Pastina	20 g
Supplements	*

* Completa Q Diet/Trovet Balance (3 g) or Essential Cat (3 g)

Maintenance recipes for active (hypoallergenic) and underactive, sterilized/neutered (hypoallergenic light) adult cats

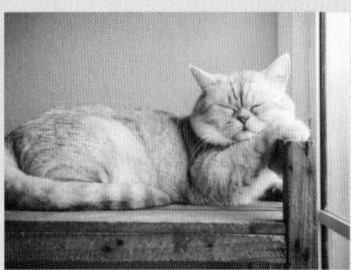

Weight: 3 kg
kcal: around 160

Ingredients	Quantity
Chicken breast	40 g
Chicken/Heart giblets, beef/pork spleen	50 g
Vegetables (pumpkin, carrot, courgette)	10 g
Supplements	*

* Completa Q Diet/Trovet Balance (2 g) or Essential Cat (2 g)

Ingredients	Quantity
Cod/Hake	110 g
Chicken/Heart giblets, beef/pork spleen	50 g
Vegetables (pumpkin, carrot, courgette)	10 g
Supplements	*

* Completa Q Diet/Trovet Balance (2 g) or Essential Cat (2 g)

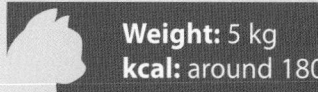

Weight: 5 kg
kcal: around 180

1

Ingredients	Quantity
Chicken breast	50 g
Chicken/Heart giblets, beef/pork spleen	50 g
Sunflower oil	1 teaspoon
Vegetables (pumpkin, carrot, courgette)	10 g
Supplements	*

* Completa Q Diet/Trovet Balance (3 g) or Essential Cat (3 g)

2

Ingredients	Quantity
Cod/Hake	120 g
Chicken/Heart giblets, beef/pork spleen	40 g
Sunflower oil	2 teaspoons
Vegetables (pumpkin, carrot, courgette)	10 g
Supplements	*

* Completa Q Diet/Trovet Balance (3 g) or Essential Cat (3 g)

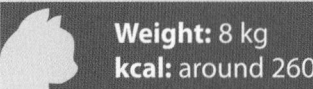

Weight: 8 kg
kcal: around 260

1

Ingredients	Quantity
Chicken breast	110 g
Chicken/Heart giblets, beef/pork spleen	50 g
Sunflower oil	2 teaspoons
Vegetables (pumpkin, carrot, courgette)	10 g
Supplements	*

* Completa Q Diet/Trovet Balance (3 g) or Essential Cat (3 g)

2

Ingredients	Quantity
Cod/Hake	160 g
Chicken/Heart giblets, beef/pork spleen	50 g
Sunflower oil	2 teaspoons
Vegetables (pumpkin, carrot, courgette)	20 g
Supplements	*

* Completa Q Diet/Trovet Balance (3 g) or Essential Cat (3 g)

Maintenance recipes for active (hypoallergenic) and underactive, sterilized/neutered (hypoallergenic light) adult cats

Weight: 3 kg
kcal: around 160

1

Ingredients	Quantity
Pork loin	100 g
Sunflower oil	1 teaspoon
Vegetables (pumpkin, carrot, courgette)	10 g
Supplements	*

Not to be administered in the period of diagnosis

* Completa Q Diet/Trovet Balance (2 g) or Essential Cat (2 g)

2

Ingredients	Quantity
Cod/Hake	180 g
Sunflower oil	1 teaspoon
Vegetables (pumpkin, carrot, courgette)	10 g
Supplements	*

Not to be administered in the period of diagnosis

* Completa Q Diet/Trovet Balance (2 g) or Essential Cat (2 g)

3

Ingredients	Quantity
Rabbit (thigh)	100 g
Sunflower oil	1 teaspoon
Vegetables (pumpkin, carrot, courgette)	10 g
Supplements	*

Not to be administered in the period of diagnosis

* Completa Q Diet/Trovet Balance (2 g) or Essential Cat (2 g)

Weight: 3 kg
kcal: around 128 (light)

1

Ingredients	Quantity
Pork loin	85 g
Vegetables (pumpkin, carrot, courgette)	10 g
Supplements	*

Not to be administered in the period of diagnosis

* Completa Q Diet/Trovet Balance (2 g) or Essential Cat (2 g)

2

Ingredients	Quantity
Cod/Hake	130 g
Sunflower oil	1 teaspoon
Vegetables (pumpkin, carrot, courgette)	10 g
Supplements	*

Not to be administered in the period of diagnosis

* Completa Q Diet/Trovet Balance (2 g) or Essential Cat (2 g)

3

Ingredients	Quantity
Rabbit (thigh)	90 g
Vegetables (pumpkin, carrot, courgette)	10 g
Supplements	*

Not to be administered in the period of diagnosis

* Completa Q Diet/Trovet Balance (2 g) or Essential Cat (2 g)

Weight: 5 kg
kcal: around 230

1

Ingredients	Quantity
Pork loin	120 g
Sunflower oil	2 teaspoons
Vegetables (pumpkin, carrot, courgette)	20 g
Supplements	*

Not to be administered in the period of diagnosis

* Completa Q Diet/Trovet Balance (3 g) or Essential Cat (3 g)

2

Ingredients	Quantity
Cod/Hake	250 g
Sunflower oil	2 teaspoons
Vegetables (pumpkin, carrot, courgette)	20 g
Supplements	*

Not to be administered in the period of diagnosis

* Completa Q Diet/Trovet Balance (3 g) or Essential Cat (3 g)

3

Ingredients	Quantity
Rabbit (thigh)	120 g
Sunflower oil	2 teaspoons
Vegetables (pumpkin, carrot, courgette)	20 g
Supplements	*

Not to be administered in the period of diagnosis

* Completa Q Diet/Trovet Balance (3 g) or Essential Cat (3 g)

Weight: 5 kg
kcal: around 180 (light)

1

Ingredients	Quantity
Pork loin	110 g
Sunflower oil	1 teaspoon
Vegetables (pumpkin, carrot, courgette)	20 g
Supplements	*

* Completa Q Diet/Trovet Balance (3 g) or Essential Cat (3 g)

Not to be administered
in the period of diagnosis

2

Ingredients	Quantity
Cod/Hake	220 g
Sunflower oil	1 teaspoon
Vegetables (pumpkin, carrot, courgette)	20 g
Supplements	*

* Completa Q Diet/Trovet Balance (3 g) or Essential Cat (3 g)

Not to be administered
in the period of diagnosis

3

Ingredients	Quantity
Rabbit (thigh)	110 g
Sunflower oil	1 teaspoon
Vegetables (pumpkin, carrot, courgette)	20 g
Supplements	*

* Completa Q Diet/Trovet Balance (3 g) or Essential Cat (3 g)

Not to be administered
in the period of diagnosis

Weight: 8 kg
kcal: around 330

1

Ingredients	Quantity
Pork loin	140 g
Pork heart and spleen	20 g
Sunflower oil	3 teaspoons
Vegetables (pumpkin, carrot, courgette)	30 g
Supplements	*

Not to be administered
in the period of diagnosis

* Completa Q Diet/Trovet Balance (3 g) or Essential Cat (3 g)

2

Ingredients	Quantity
Cod/Hake	270 g
Sunflower oil	4 teaspoons
Vegetables (pumpkin, carrot, courgette)	40 g
Supplements	*

Not to be administered
in the period of diagnosis

* Completa Q Diet/Trovet Balance (3 g) or Essential Cat (3 g)

3

Ingredients	Quantity
Rabbit (thigh)	170 g
Sunflower oil	3 teaspoons
Vegetables (pumpkin, carrot, courgette)	30 g
Supplements	*

Not to be administered
in the period of diagnosis

* Completa Q Diet/Trovet Balance (3 g) or Essential Cat (3 g)

Weight: 8 kg
kcal: around 260 (light)

1

Ingredients	Quantity
Pork loin	130 g
Pork heart and spleen	20 g
Sunflower oil	1 teaspoon
Vegetables (pumpkin, carrot, courgette)	30 g
Supplements	*

Not to be administered
in the period of diagnosis

* Completa Q Diet/Trovet Balance (3 g) or Essential Cat (3 g)

2

Ingredients	Quantity
Cod/Hake	260 g
Sunflower oil	3 teaspoons
Vegetables (pumpkin, carrot, courgette)	40 g
Supplements	*

Not to be administered
in the period of diagnosis

* Completa Q Diet/Trovet Balance (3 g) or Essential Cat (3 g)

3

Ingredients	Quantity
Rabbit (thigh)	160 g
Sunflower oil	1 teaspoon
Vegetables (pumpkin, carrot, courgette)	30 g
Supplements	*

Not to be administered
in the period of diagnosis

* Completa Q Diet/Trovet Balance (3 g) or Essential Cat (3 g)

Maintenance recipes for active (BARF) and underactive, sterilized/neutered (BARF light) adult cats

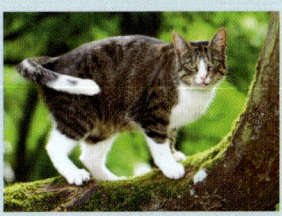

Weight: 3 kg
kcal: around 160

Ingredients	Quantity
Beef	60 g
Beef heart, spleen, kidneys, lungs, liver	40 g
Sunflower oil	1 teaspoon
Vegetables (pumpkin, carrot, courgette)	10 g
Beer yeast (deactivated)	1 g
Supplements	*

* Completa Q Diet/Trovet Balance (2 g) or Essential Cat (2 g)

Weight: 3 kg
kcal: around 128 (light)

Ingredients	Quantity
Beef	50 g
Beef heart, spleen, kidneys, lungs, liver	40 g
Vegetables (pumpkin, carrot, courgette)	10 g
Beer yeast (deactivated)	1 g
Supplements	*

* Completa Q Diet/Trovet Balance (2 g) or Essential Cat (2 g)

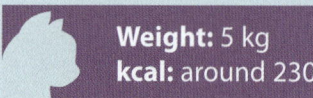

Weight: 5 kg
kcal: around 230

Ingredients	Quantity
Beef	100 g
Beef heart, spleen, kidneys, lungs, liver	50 g
Sunflower oil	1 teaspoon
Vegetables (pumpkin, carrot, courgette)	20 g
Beer yeast (deactivated)	1 g
Supplements	*

* Completa Q Diet/Trovet Balance (3 g) or Essential Cat (3 g)

Weight: 5 kg
kcal: around 180 (light)

Ingredients	Quantity
Beef	70 g
Beef heart, spleen, kidneys, lungs, liver	40 g
Sunflower oil	1 teaspoon
Vegetables (pumpkin, carrot, courgette)	10 g
Beer yeast (deactivated)	1 g
Supplements	*

* Completa Q Diet/Trovet Balance (3 g) or Essential Cat (3 g)

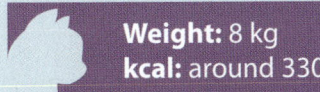

Weight: 8 kg
kcal: around 330

Ingredients	Quantity
Beef	120 g
Beef heart, spleen, kidneys, lungs, liver	60 g
Sunflower oil	2 teaspoons
Vegetables (pumpkin, carrot, courgette)	30 g
Beer yeast (deactivated)	1 g
Supplements	*

* Completa Q Diet/Trovet Balance (3 g) or Essential Cat (3 g)

Weight: 8 kg
kcal: around 260 (light)

Ingredients	Quantity
Beef	90 g
Beef heart, spleen, kidneys, lungs, liver	50 g
Sunflower oil	2 teaspoons
Vegetables (pumpkin, carrot, courgette)	30 g
Beer yeast (deactivated)	1 g
Supplements	*

* Completa Q Diet/Trovet Balance (3 g) or Essential Cat (3 g)

Chapter 6

Alimentary behavior

From the bowl to the mind

Raimondo Colangeli

OBJECTIVES OF THIS CHAPTER
• Understand the ethological aspect of alimentary behavior • Evaluate alimentary behavior in the context of the diagnosis of behavioral pathologies

Alimentary behavior must be analyzed not only in its physiological component, but also in its mental aspect, therefore from both an emotional and cognitive point of view.

The novelties that emerged in neuroscience and PNEI (*psychoneuroendocrineimmunology* is the science that studies the interactions between the central, endocrine and immune systems, as well as their effect on human and animal behavior) lead us to the abandonment of a vision which was focused solely on the study of specific aspect, in this case the nutritional one, to broaden our evaluation to the whole organism and mind.

The primary function of behavior is the adaptation to changes in the environment (external and internal); behavior becomes pathological when it loses its plasticity, therefore its adaptive abilities.

We will therefore analyze the alimentary behavior in different aspects:

- neurophysiology and ethology;
- social prerogative as regards the management of food resources;
- predatory aggression behavior;
- behavioral semiology: signs and symptoms that direct us to a differential diagnosis between an organic pathology and behavioral pathologies.

Neurophysiology and ethology

Alimentary behavior is defined as a set of motor acts performed by the animal with the aim of researching, accepting and ingesting elements recognized as food and intended to feed on them. It is a complex system that goes beyond eating (and drinking) and relies on external factors (stimuli present in the external environment) and internal factors (metabolism and neurotransmitters). In fact, in a current neuroscientific vision, we speak of interconnection between the hypothalamic system and the sensory system, between the limbic system and the prefrontal cortex, where cognitive areas interact with the areas that govern emotions.

Therefore, we can better understand why the ingestion of the food is linked to the congruence between smell and taste, and how the palatability varies regarding to the origin of the food (amino acid receptors) and to the novelty of food, which is strictly individual (see below, definition of coprophagia): this leads to *neophilia* (introduction of new nutritional elements in the diet) or to *alimentary neophobia* (survival regarding to the toxic effects) (Box 6.1).

As for the influence of sex hormones on alimentary behavior, we know that both estrogen and testosterone tend to decrease appetite; in fact, we note an increase in weight in sterilized animals due to increased hunger, metabolic changes, reduced physical activity and, last but not least, emotional factors of the owners (guilt associated with incorrect food rituals).

In the wild, wild canids ingest a large quantity of food in a short time, following the capture of prey and the dissection through biting; a wild canid can ingest up to 20% of its weight in food, but it can also eat every 3 days; this is due to the uncertainty of the capture of the prey, the difficulty to store the food and the competition with other animals.

In the wild, dogs feed during the day and just a few times. Perhaps this is the reason behind the popular belief or for convenience, that owners used to give food to their dogs only once a day (with possible gastric pathologies: gastritis or vulnerability to GDV (gastric dilatation volvulus, gastric dilatation/torsion syndrome).

BOX 6.1 THE GARCIA EFFECT OR LEARNED GUSTATIVE REVERSE

John Garcia, an ethologist at Harvard Medical School, in the 1950s carried out an experiment with rats which proved to be very interesting in the gustatory field.

Garcia fed the rats with a sweet liquid and, subsequently, gave them a substance that caused vomiting or nausea for a short period: it immediately emerged that, even after a single experiment, the rats that had received that substance always avoided the sweet stimulus.

It proves that learning the aversion of a flavor is the result of a particular function of associative memory (based in the hippocampus and amygdala), which is common to all animal species. A single negative experience is enough to compromise the attitude towards a certain food: this instinct may seem no longer necessary for pets, but in nature an animal cannot afford to slowly learn the potential deadly effect of a food.

The indication, as already described, of a division into two but also into three meals a day for a lifetime is useful to prevent the aforementioned pathologies, as well as the anxious pathologies with gastroenteric manifestations. Returning to the feeding of dogs in nature, it is not uncommon to notice them search for grass and ingesting it: this behavior often seems a sort of "self-phytotherapy", since, in addition to promoting gastric emptying or intestinal evacuation, the choice of particular species of plants is part of the self-medication of indigenous human populations who cannot access Western medicine.

Coprophagia is a highly unwanted behavior on the part of the owners, since it is not a pleasure to receive an affectionate lick on the face from their dog after they have swallowed feces. Coprophagia is a physiological and ancestral alimentary behavior: the mother, in the first days of the puppies' lives, when neurological control of the sphincter is still absent, at the end of the feed turns the puppy in a supine position and licks the genital poles, favoring the release of feces (of milky content) and urine, which are ingested to keep the "nest" clean.

Continued on the next page

Continued from the previous page

So, the feces of other animals are palatable for smell and taste, linked to the presence of high protein concentrations and their characteristics.

Often it happens that the owners tell of a puppy that eats its feces exclusively at home: this can be linked to the learning of not to defecate in the house, previously implemented with punishments by the owners; in this case, the puppy eliminates the evidence by ingesting the stool and it hides to urinate (Figure 6.1).

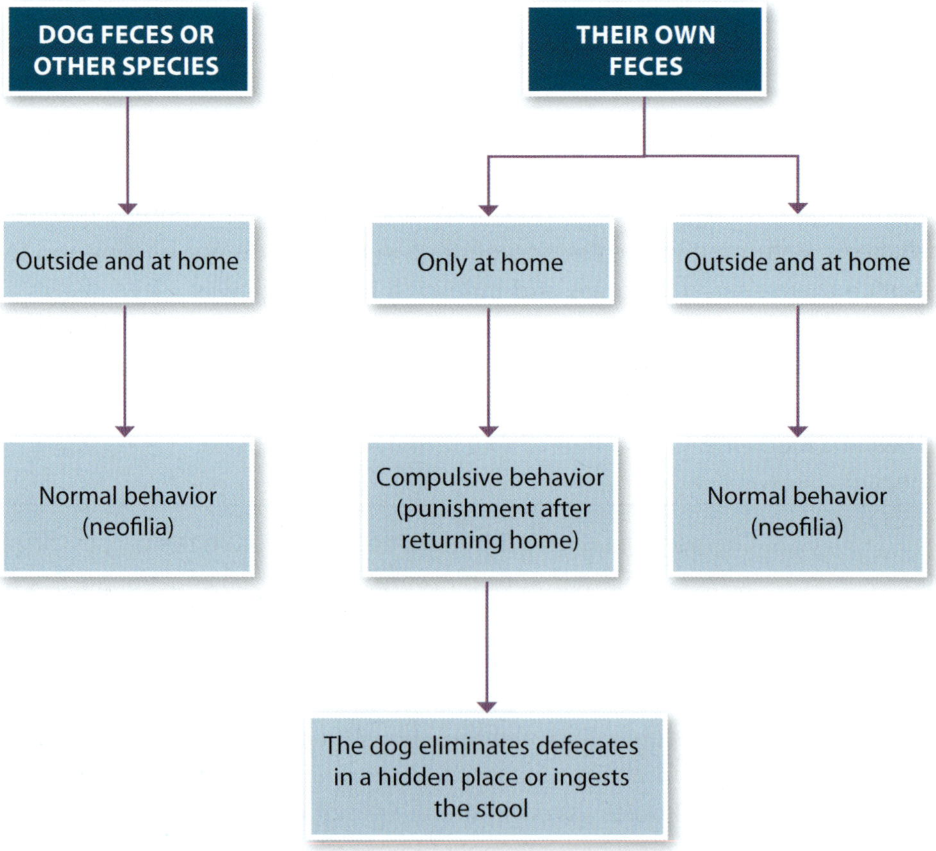

DOG FECES OR OTHER SPECIES	THEIR OWN FECES	
Outside and at home	Only at home	Outside and at home
Normal behavior (neofilia)	Compulsive behavior (punishment after returning home)	Normal behavior (neofilia)

The dog eliminates defecates in a hidden place or ingests the stool

■ **FIGURE 6.1** Coprophagia in the puppy.

Social prerogative regarding the management of food resources

The food resource falls within one of the four social prerogatives, together with the management of the territory, the management of the reproductive aspect and, above all, the management of social contacts, also called control of the initiative. Therefore, investigating alimentary behavior allows us to obtain information on the relational aspect within the human-dog family group.

However, we must quickly clear the field of obsolete and misleading concepts related to the notion of alpha dog and hierarchies based on dominance (and therefore submission), explaining the evolution of the concept of hierarchy. The alpha wolf/dog is a figure looming in our imagination and a notion deeply rooted and conveyed in our thoughts. Why? The idea of the alpha wolf comes from Rudolph Schenkel, a scholar of animal behavior, who in 1947 published a revolutionary study for its time, called *Expressions Studies on Wolves*, resulting from the observation of wolves in the zoo of Basel, Switzerland. He defined the sociology of the wolf, then superimposed it on the sociability of the domestic dog. In his research, Schenkel had identified two primary wolves in a pack: a male and a female "running wolves". He had described them as "first in the pack" and had also noticed "violent rivalry" between individual members regarding the management of social prerogatives, particularly those that linked to food management.

A key problem with Schenkel's research on wolves was that, although it constituted the first close study of wolves, it did not involve any study of wolves in nature. Schenkel had studied two wolf packs that lived in captivity, but his research has remained the main source of wolf behavior for decades. Later, other researchers would conduct their studies of captive wolves and publish similar results on dominance-submission relationships within captive wolf packs. In addition, the notion of "alpha wolf" was largely reinforced by the 1970 book by wildlife biologist L. David Mech, The Wolf: *The Ecology and Behavior of an Endangered Species*.

In more recent years, animal behavioral scholars, including Mech, have spent more and more time studying wolves in the wild and the observed behaviors have turned out to be different from those observed by Schenkel and other researchers in wolves living in zoos.

In 1999, Mech published the article "Alpha Status, Dominance, and Division of Labor in Wolf Packs" in the *Canadian Journal of Zoology*.

This study is considered by many to be a breakthrough in understanding the structure of wolf packs. «The concept of the alpha wolf that governs a group of conspecifics of a similar age», writes Mech in the 1999 article, «is particularly misleading». He explains that his studies on wild wolves have found that wolves live in families: two parents together with their younger pups. Wolves do not have an innate sense of rank, they are not born dominant or submissive.

Nobody has "won" a group leader role, but parents can assert dominance over their offspring by virtue of being parents. It is the paradigmatic transition from the dominance hierarchy, based on competition, to the family hierarchy, based on the collaboration and referentiality of the parental figures and adults present in the family group. The younger wolf does not overthrow the "alpha" to become the leader of the pack.

Mech highlighted that the typical herd is a family in which the parents lead the group's activities by dividing the tasks: the females are mainly involved in caring for and defending the puppies, the males are busy procuring food by alternately dividing the leadership according to the case. The term "leadership" indicates situations in which a wolf controls and directs the behavior of other individuals, choosing the direction of the move, when and where to stop to rest and whether or not to chase a prey. If the prey that is caught is large enough, all members of the pack, regardless of rank, eat together, while «[...] if the food is scarce, the puppies will take precedence».

Mech also writes: «[...] the attempt to apply the information derived from the observation of herds consisting of elements without any kinship link to natural herds, has contributed to creating considerable confusion. Such an approach is analogous to wanting to draw conclusions about the family behavior of men by studying the behavior of people living in a refugee camp».

However, the outdated idea of the "alpha wolf" still catches on in an area of the real world: dog training.

The idea of the herd and hierarchy is often taken to the extreme; dog owners are provided with a list of rules on how to maintain alpha status in all aspects of their relationship: don't let your dog go through the door before you; don't let him win a tug of war game; don't let it eat before you. Some instructors, even successful ones, even encourage acts of physical domination that can be dangerous for owners to perform. These indications, for the most part, derive from the old studies on wolves mentioned above and erroneously establish that one must be in constant competition with one's dogs for the position of the leader of the pack.

 So how does this new information apply in the food management of the dog included in the family group? The concept of food hierarchy is outdated, where the mother prevents the puppy from approaching the food to define its lower status, a behavior that is later taken up by the owner who eats before the dog or does not give him food from the table. This aspect does not determine leadership.

When we find ourselves in the presence of a behavioral pathology called competitive relationship disorder, from the food point of view we observe a dog that manifests:

1. A pressing and repeated request for food, jumping on people until it leads to aggression or theft of food from the table or from kitchen surfaces.
2. Food theft from the table or from the kitchen counter.
3. Snarl, if family members, strangers or other dogs approach the bowl or found/stolen food; the snarl can be with your mouth closed or open (linked to the fluctuation of the arousal, i.e. the level of impulsiveness of the subject); the dog has a rigid posture and stops taking food; if the intruder does not stop, it can trigger the attack with a bite. It is important to distinguish this behavior of competitive aggression for food from the defense of food (linked to a shortage of food or, more often, to the difficulty of reaching food if it is given to puppies in a single bowl before adoption: the less enterprising feeds with difficulty). In this case the dog continues to eat avidly, not by lifting the muzzle from the bowl but by continuing to growl (in this circumstance the puppy's confidence in the owner must be increased by adding food from time to time during meals).
4. Capricious appetite, otherwise called "the tasting dog": is another way to manifest a competition on the management of food. A woman told me about the difficulties in feeding her 2-year-old male Yorkshire Terrier: «My dog wants to eat only twice-ground beef from the butcher in the square and not from the one next door to my flat, otherwise he won't eat». Often, the concept "I prepare food for you and therefore I love you" and "you love me if you eat what I prepared for you" results in a ritual that can be dysfunctional in the relationship between the owner and the dog.
5. Acceleration of food intake in front of others, while shy dogs may not approach the bowl and not eat if one or more family members are present.

BOX 6.2 THE REWARD

In the education of a puppy, in training courses as in the rehabilitative intervention of a dog suffering from behavioral pathologies, food is often used as "primary reinforcement". According to learning techniques, using a reward/treat allows you to increase the frequency of an already acquired behavior or to express a new behavior compared to another unwanted one. However, from a nutritional point of view, we must choose a qualitatively correct food: too many dog professionals use extremely energetic foods or too fatty ones (for example sausages and cheese) and in exaggerated quantities. In addition to representing a nutritional error, these reinforcements pre-eminently activate the reward circuit of the dopamine neurotransmitter system, which if on one hand feeds pleasure and gratification, on the other it can lead to the phenomenon of dependence in the cases of abuse.

For this reason, it is appropriate to use simultaneously, and above all, a "social" reward that activates the serotonergic system, which are the affectionate attitudes such as caresses, a sweet and fulfilling voice to express one's satisfaction with respect to the behavior of the dog. As explained with neuroscientific concepts by Robert Lustig in his book *The Hacking of the American Mind*, pleasure is triggered by dopamine ("I want more and more"), while happiness is produced by serotonin ("I am satisfied with what I got ").

A recommendation for owners who must reward their dog which, however, presents intolerance/allergies and follows an excluding diet: there are rewards of different brands with monoproteinic content equal to that chosen in the diet; alternatively, you can buy fresh food and, divide it into small pieces, dry it or, more simply, in the oven at 60-70° C for about 2 hours.

Predatory aggression behavior

Unlike other aggression behaviors, i.e. competition, irritation, fear, territorial and maternal behavior, which have a communicative function (I threaten or bite you to communicate something), predatory aggression behavior has a function associated with the motivation of the food. It is a behavior that is defined as instinctive and, in fact, is produced by the stimulation of the lateral hypothalamus, therefore from the phylogenetically older part of the brain, with connection between hypothalamic regions and centers of satiety. It is a behavior that consists of a sequence divided into three phases:

1. **Initial or appetitive phase:** the waiting phase is generally reinforced by a hypoglycemia that increases the alertness of the dog, with the result of making it receptive to the slightest jerky movement present in the surrounding environment: an animal becomes prey at the moment it moves.
2. **Central phase:** the killing of the prey with dissection and consummation bites. Consumption and predation, however, do not go hand in hand: in fact, the presence of numerous prey in a closed place can trigger predation in sated subjects: it happened that one morning a marten was found asleep in a chicken coop, exhausted by the killing of all the hens, of which it had consumed only one.
3. **Terminal or arrest phase** (calming or inhibition enhanced by hyperglycaemia).

However, instinct alone does not allow the dog to perform: the experience acquired, training and/or imitation of an expert adult dog must be added.

In addition, predatory behavior must be divided according to the type of prey:

- small-sized prey: generally it is an individual predation, in which the dog jumps on the prey with its feet close together, falling with the front legs to immobilize it; then the prey is grabbed with the jaws and shaken violently, fracturing the cervical spine. This behavior is often performed by adult dogs and puppies in their games. It is an absolutely acceptable predatory play behavior on an inanimate object, as opposed to the "push and pull" between owner and dog;
- large prey: it is a group predation, in which strategy and collaboration are fundamental for success. The prey is chosen and, when it flees, the chase starts, followed by immobilization and death by dissection.

A fundamental characteristic of predatory behavior is the insufficient or absent interaction with subjects of its own species and of other species, which the dog acquires during the socialization period, indicatively between the 30th and 120th day of life. This explains why the rehabilitation intervention has poor, if not zero, results; prevention is the only way forward. An early and repeated knowledge of their conspecifics should lead the dog to a "generalized" socialization with all the other dogs. However, this is not entirely true, since the degree of socialization also depends on the dog's self-control and emotional stability.

In addition, acting in a pack can trigger the pursuit and, sometimes, the injury (in the most serious cases the killing) of small dogs, which become "prey". On the contrary, interspecific socialization is defined as "partial" (limited for example to animals in the family and not to external ones) or "categorized" (as far as humans are concerned, having had experience with the category of adults does not mean knowing the category of infants, different from the category of children, adolescents, the elderly, foreigners, disabled people with uncertain gait, those in uniforms such as postmen, nuns, soldiers, etc.). Therefore, the main prevention that we can implement, is a positive and an early experience with the various types of "humans".

Behavioral semiology: signs and symptoms that direct us to the differential diagnosis between organic pathologies and behavioral pathologies

Beyond the evaluation of an organic pathology which is responsible for a change in appetite, the characteristics of the latter can direct us towards a mental pathological state and, therefore, towards the diagnosis of a behavioral pathology, in which the rehabilitation intervention can be accompanied with supportive pharmacological/nutraceutical/pheromonal therapy.

- *Anorexia*: is present in acute depressive states. An example can be observed at the time of the puppy's detachment and insertion into the new social group; often the owners tell of an animal that does not move in the new house, does not explore, does not eat, does not eliminate. This situation is incompatible with life and cannot last long, but thanks to domestication the dog quickly puts in place a secondary attachment to the adopting group of humans (or other present dogs) that replaces the maternal figure and that of the initial group. Another example is the loss of a reference figure within the social group (a figure of the family or a group of present dogs) by death or simply by removal.
- *Hyporexia*: the decrease in appetite can occur partially, depending on the context (at home or outside, Figure 6.2).
- *Dysorexia* or *fluctuation of appetite*: this condition, that is an alternation of periods of bulimia with periods of hyporexia, can occur especially in the chronic depressive syndrome of an elderly dog, which is accompanied by other symptoms, including altered sleep with difficulty in the falling

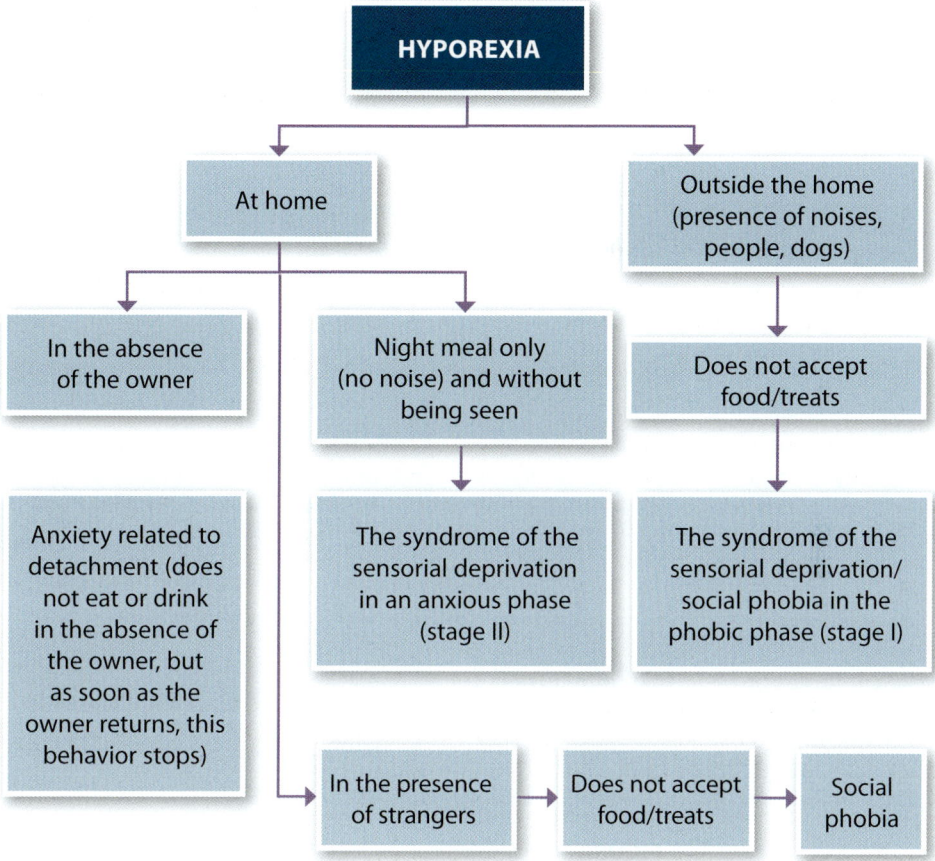

FIGURE 6.2 Decreased appetite: hyporexia.

asleep and sudden nocturnal awakenings.

- *Bulimia* (from the Greek *boulimía*, "ox hunger"): this defines an excessive voracity linked to organic pathologies such as diabetes or behavioral pathologies; in human medicine it is called *bulimia nervosa* and, together with anorexia, is part of the disorders of alimentary behavior. It is important not to associate the concept of bulimic hyperphagia with that of the obesity: its characteristics are the increase in food intake with permanent searching for food and a progressive decrease in the state of contentment after ingestion (stereotype). In fact, depending on the age of onset of this symptom in the life of the dog, different behavioral pathologies can be identified (Figure 6.3).

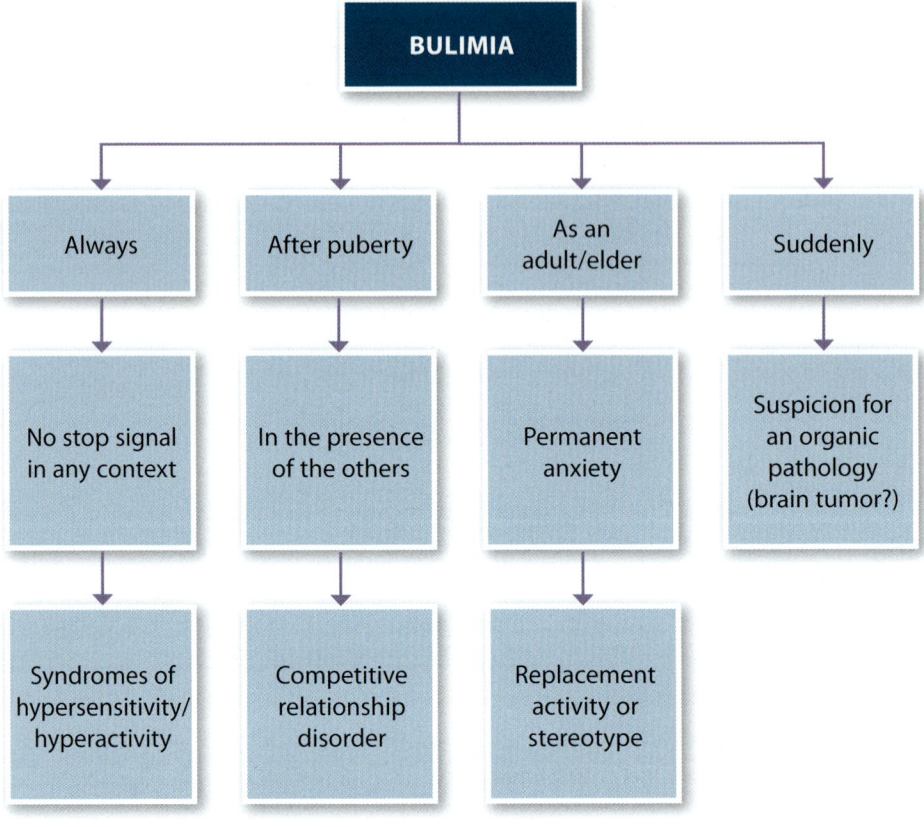

■ **FIGURE 6.3** Pathological voracity: bulimia.

Alimentary behavior of the cat

Even the cat, which is now part of the social group of humans on a permanent basis, has changed its alimentary behavior over time. It was born as a mainly nocturnal solitary predator: formidable hunter of small prey such as rodents and birds, it was used by the Egyptians and other people in antiquity as a defender of food reserves (fossil finds in China, dated 5600 B.C.E., demonstrate a diet based on rodents and millet). With the acquisition of the status of pet, its life, in many cases, takes place within the home, without the need to obtain food.

At home, unfortunately, feeding is often far from the ethological characteristics of the cat: in nature, the predatory behavior of small prey is the only way for this animal to get food. But out of 15-20 attempts, only a few are successful: this means making 5-10 small meals a day. The cat, therefore, is not a "small dog" (as owners often think) that should be fed twice a day, but it is far more preferable to feed it five and perhaps several times a day in small quantities, which based on your choice might be wet, dry or home prepared foods. The dry food, being less palatable, can be left available for the cat, but this depends on the characteristics of its appetite (similar to those that we saw in the paragraph on the dog).

From a social point of view, the cat's alimentary behavior does not have hierarchical values: in a group of cats the first one that arrives, eats (but it is always better to divide the meal into several bowls), without aggression. Kittens who have had difficulty in obtaining food can demonstrate a defense of food by covering the bowl with their bodies and moving their neighbor with their paws, but it is a rare event.

The cat, this stranger

The minor knowledge on the cat's behavioral needs leads the owner to interpret its requests incorrectly, making even serious nutritional errors for the animal's health. An example is the return home of the owner: the cat, who often stays alone for many hours in a house with little or no "environmental enrichment", runs towards the owner on their arrival and, rubbing on their legs and meowing, invites playful interaction (chasing toys or pampering). This request, however, is often interpreted as a request for food, reinforced by a sense of guilt for having left the cat alone for a long time.

And then what? The cat is rewarded by feeding it with food that is often "prohibited": the result is less physical activity and a repeated request for food when the owner returns home (with dopaminergic gratification), with a consequent tendency to obesity.

Frequently the cat is supercharged, with evident hyperphagia and an absence of satiety. The chosen diet must also be modulated in the day and divided into several meals. Many owners are absent for several hours during the day: a piece of good advice is to use an automatic dispenser with opening of the compartments at set times.

References

Cerquetella M, Rossi G, Spaterna A, Tesei B et al. Is irritable bowel syndrome also present in dogs? *Tierarztl Prax Ausg K Kleintiere Heimtiere.* 2018;46(3):176-180.

European Pet Food Industry Federation. *Nutritional Guidelines for Complete and Complementary Pet Food for Cats and Dogs.* FEDIAF, Brussels, 2019.

Fascetti AJ, Delaney SJ (Eds.). *Applied Veterinary Clinical Nutrition.* Wiley-Blackwell, Hoboken, 2012.

Hand MS, Thatcher CD, Remillard RL et al. (Eds.). *Small Animal Clinical Nutrition,* 5th ed. Mark Morris Institute, Topeka, 2010.

Lecoindre P, Gaschen FP. Chronic idiopathic large bowel diarrhea in the dog. *Vet Clin North Am Small Anim Pract.* 2011;41(2):447-56.

Leib MS. Treatment of chronic idiopathic large-bowel diarrhea in dogs with a highly digestible diet and soluble fiber: a retrospective review of 37 cases. *J Vet Intern Med.* 2000;14(1):27-32.

McDonald P, Edwards RA, Greenhalgh JFD et al. (Eds.). *Animal Nutrition,* 7th ed. Pearson Education, Harlow, 2011.

Olivry T, Mueller RS, Prélaud P. Critically appraised topic on adverse food reactions of companion animals (1): duration of elimination diets. *BMC Vet Res.* 2015;11:225.

Outerbridge CA. *Nutritional Management of Skin Diseases.* In: Fascetti AJ, Delaney SJ (Eds.). *Applied Veterinary Clinical Nutrition.* Wiley-Blackwell, Hoboken, 2012.

Singh B. Psyllium as therapeutic and drug delivery agent. *Int J Pharm.* 2007; 334(1-2):1-14.

Verlinden A, Hesta M, Millet S, Janssens GP. Food allergy in dogs and cats: a review. *Crit Rev Food Sci Nutr.* 2006;46(3):259-273.

Villaverde C, Hervera M. *Adverse food reactions in small animals.* In: Chan DL (Ed.). *Nutritional Management of Hospitalized Small Animals.* Wiley & Sons Ltd., Chichester, 2015.